WAKE-UP CALL

Caitlin Press Inc.
8100 Alderwood Road,
Halfmoon Bay, BC V0N 1Y1
www.caitlin-press.com

Cover Photograph: ist2_8792921
Edited by Erin Schpofer.
Printed in Canada

Caitlin Press Inc. acknowledges financial support from the Government of Canada through the Book Publishing Industry Development Program and the Canada
Council for the Arts, and from the Province of British Columbia through the British Columbia Arts Council and the Book Publisher's Tax Credit.

 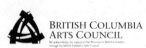

Canada Council for the Arts **Conseil des Arts du Canada** BRITISH COLUMBIA ARTS COUNCIL

Library and Archives Canada Cataloguing in Publication

Haynes, Sterling

    Wake-up call : tales from a frontier

doctor / Sterling Haynes.

ISBN 978-1-894759-44-1

    1. Haynes, Sterling. 2. Medicine, Rural—Anecdotes.

3. Physicians—Canada—Biography. I. Title.

R464.H395A3 2010   610.92   C2010-900679-8

WAKE-UP CALL

TALES FROM A
FRONTIER DOCTOR

STERLING HAYNES

CAITLIN PRESS

I dedicate this book to my mother, Elizabeth Sterling Haynes

Table of Contents

INTRODUCTION

Laughter has helped me through many difficult times in life and medicine. A good chuckle can put things in perspective. When I was seventy and in retirement, I had a left hemisphere stroke and my brain became rearranged. It was then that I became more creative and perhaps funnier. My creative right side took over and I started to write poetry and humour. I was left with a partially paralyzed right foot but a writer's creative right brain. I think I got the better end of the deal, but then I may be prejudiced.

The funny memories from my life as a medical doctor became hilarious and the sad, melancholy memories looked less bleak. I started writing about my years as a doctor and found that magazines and newspapers were interested in my stories. After my stroke I wrote a poem that exemplifies my change in life philosophy.

Life No. 2
"We write to taste life twice."
—Anais Nin
i write to taste
life twice and

have a second
belly laugh

along the way

After my residency in Oakland, California, my wife, Jessie, and I loaded our infant daughter, Elizabeth, and all our possessions in our old Volkswagen bug and headed for the frontier town of Williams Lake, British Columbia. "Willie's Puddle" was a busy town of a few thousand people. Four doctors serviced the town and the huge, rugged area surrounding it known as the Chilcotin. The local forty-bed hospital was old and dilapidated but it met the needs of the loggers, ranchers, miners, locals and First Nations people. Three of our daughters, Melissa, Jocelyn and Leslie were born there. When I first arrived in Williams Lake all the hospital rooms, except (thank god) the operating room and case room, were lit with 40-watt bulbs, making medical examinations very difficult. Under these conditions I delivered hundreds of babies, performed emergency surgery and gave anaesthetics. Besides poor lighting, another problem we faced was heating: when people left the front door of the hospital open in the winter the furnace would blow out. This could be disastrous if there were newborns in the nursery.

We worked long hours, made house calls, went out with the ambulance and flew to remote accident sites in the Chilcotin. Before socialized healthcare was introduced, we would sometimes receive payment in-kind because the miners and stump ranchers often had little money set aside with which to pay a doctor. I was paid in hinds of beef, lamb and moose and in bags of potatoes and turnips, which I hauled to the cold storage room in my basement. On one occasion, a big game guide brought me a four-point buck in payment for delivering his first son; he left the dressed carcass in the centre of my waiting room.

My first practice in Williams Lake taught me how to be a real doctor.

I learned to improvise and to look at all sides of a problem. I learned compassion, patience and humour. These attributes stood me in good stead when we moved to Kamloops six years later and then on to rural Marion, Alabama. By then I knew about most Canadian diseases but in Alabama I had to learn about sickle-cell anemia, black skin dermatology, the treatment of frequent gunshot wounds and extensive straight-razor cuts. My patients were generally poor, kind and considerate. I was their Doc and they trusted me to do the right thing.

Many illnesses now looked after by specialists were at that time looked after by rural doctors. Many of my stories are funny but some speak to the various medical tragedies that humans endure and to the racial injustices of the time.

Looking back on my thirty-seven years in medicine, it shaped my life, but I wouldn't have missed it for the world.

Beginnings

Mother Blood

In 1909 Karl Landsteiner, a Viennese medical doctor, discovered different types of human blood and classified the differences into A, B, AB and O groups. About eleven years later, in New York, he collaborated with Drs. Levine and Weiner and discovered the Rh factor of blood. These discoveries led to the development of methods for safe blood transfusions that were then used to treat people injured in the Spanish civil war. Dr. Landsteiner won the Nobel Prize in Physiology or Medicine in 1930 for his discovery of human blood groups.

After the Japanese air attack on Pearl Harbor, December 7, 1941, thousands of American sailors and marines were in need of blood transfusions. December 7 was also my mother's birthday and on this particular Sunday my mother needed blood transfusions as well.

Mother, at age forty-three, had developed cancer of the womb and had received preoperative radium inserts at the University of Alberta Hospital, in Edmonton, to contain her malignancy.

On the previous Friday Mother had undergone a hysterectomy and she had lost a significant amount of blood and was very weak. On December 7 it was determined that in order for mother to survive she would need two massive blood transfusions. My sister Shirley and I were both Group O, Rh positive as was my mother. The crossmatch showed that our blood would be compatible with hers.

At two o'clock in the afternoon I was skating at the Garneau community ice rink in Edmonton with my friends to the tune of "I've Got a Lovely Bunch of Coconuts." Halfway through the skate the music cut off and the announcer said, "The United States has declared war on Japan. The number of American naval and marine casualties at Pearl Harbor was large and many US ships were destroyed." Just after that grim news my father appeared outside the fence of the skating rink. He was ashen in appearance—I knew something was wrong at home.

"Sterling," he said, "change your skates right away. Your mother is critically sick in the surgical ward in the hospital and we need you immediately. You have to tranfuse your mother with your blood. We need at least a quart of blood from you and another quart from Shirley."

The illegal tag game I was playing with the Sawatsky twins and my best friend Percy came to an end. I let them know that I had to go to the hospital. My mother was sick and for the first time, at the age of fourteen, my mother needed me.

Rushing home I saw that Dad had got the car out of the garage and had it parked on Eighty-fourth Avenue. Our tires crunched through snow and ice as we drove towards the University of Alberta Hospital.

Dr. Horner, Mother's surgeon-gynecologist, was waiting at the top of the steps. He guided us both into a small operating room theatre that was divided by a raised six-foot stage, which contained a stretcher, numerous lengths of glass partitions and a long piece of rubber tubing. I climbed the stairs to the raised platform. I shed my warm clothes and peeled down my long winter underwear from my chest and then was instructed to lie on the stretcher. My mother lay pale and motionless on a stretcher six feet below me.

"Dad, is Mom okay? She'll be okay, Dr. Horner? Won't she?"

"Yes, son, she'll be okay once she gets the blood into her. You pay strict attention to what Dr. Horner tells you."

"Sterling, I am going to put a large needle into your arm and we are going to run blood from your arm to your mother's arm. Your mother is very tired now but as soon as the blood is given she will perk up a bit. The blood will flow by gravity. You must lie still for about an hour. Do you understand?" said Dr. Horner.

"Yes sir, I understand, I won't move a muscle. I'm pretty tough. Hope Mom will be okay soon."

My blood started to flow down the rubber tubing into my mother's arm; the tubing looked like a massive umbilical vein.

After about an hour Mother seemed a little more restless and spoke to me. "Are you alright, Sterling? You know, I seem to feel better already."

"Yeah, I'm okay, Mom—I've got lots of blood. I'm a big strong kid. When I'm finished here Shirley is waiting to come in and give you more blood. I guess they'll hook things up to Shirl's forearm vein and fill you full of more blood."

The nurses and Dr. Horner came in and my sister Shirley lay down on the stretcher while I stood beside it. When Shirley was in place I was disconnected and the needle was removed. The long rubber tubing was then hooked up to a new needle in my older sister's arm. I felt a bit light-headed at first but Dr. Horner told me that this was to be expected as I'd given my Mother over three pints of blood. He told me I would be fine to go back to school the next day.

My dad and my sister stayed with Mother at the hospital. I was told to walk home and get supper ready and they'd be back around seven o'clock that evening.

"Your mom will be okay now. She has your blood and now your sister's to help her recover. It was a great birthday present," said Dr. Horner.

I remember walking back home along the roadway at dusk. People were putting their house lights on and the bulbs cast a yellow glow to the long shadows. I kicked the large frozen horse droppings we called "buns," left from horse-pulled bread wagons and milk carts. I knew Mom would be better now with new blood and would soon be home from the hospital. I started to sing and dance as I slid, kicked "buns" and walked along the icy and snow-covered road—"I've got a lovely bunch of coconuts, big ones, thick ones, some as big as your head."

DR. HARRY

On a sunny August day in 1938 I was walking and humming a Winnie the Pooh Bear song, "Nobody Knows Tiddly Pom," and not paying much attention. I'd been swimming in Edmonton's south side pool and my eyes were red from chlorine. Not seeing well and being awkward to begin with—I was a fat little kid—I fell scrambling in a public rock garden and broke and dislocated my left elbow.

My eleven-year-old chum, Bill, saw that my arm looked "kind of funny" and ran across the street and asked a solid citizen to drive us home. Each bump in the gravel road caused me to let out a howl.

At home, my mother phoned the office of Dr. Harry Weinlos and his nurse told her to take me to the Misericordia Hospital. Dr. Harry, a prominent Alberta surgeon, would see me when I got there. I was told not to eat or drink anything. Mother called a cab and took me to the hospital.

At the Mizz Dr. Harry appeared. He was a short, stocky man with a small black moustache, a kind face and large, strong-looking hands. He wore small rimless glasses and behind the lenses he had bright twinkly eyes. This was the first of many meetings with this compassionate man. Over the years, Dr. Harry became my doctor, mentor and hero.

"Well, Sterling, you have painful-looking elbow. We'll have to take an x-ray and then Dr. Adamson will put a mask over your face and put you to sleep with some smelly stuff—it's called a 1–2–3 gas and you'll waken with your elbow fixed and no more pain. It's as simple as 1–2–3."

"Thanks, Dr. Weinlos, I'll try and be good but my arm really hurts."

Even now I can remember Dr. Adamson putting the mask over my face and dripping some 1–2–3 liquid on the cloth mesh as I struggled to breathe. Years later I would learn that the metal mask covered in layers of cloth was called a Schimmelbusch mask. The 1–2–3 liquid dripped onto the mask was comprised of chloroform, alcohol and ether. This very potent mixture quickly put me under. I remember waking up in the kids' ward vomiting and smelling ether but my left arm didn't hurt. My fracture dislocation had been relocated. The next day Dr. Weinlos sent me home in a cast with a sling. There was no physiotherapy in Edmonton at that time; the only rehabilitation was provided by Dr. Harry himself.

After eight weeks Dr. Harry cut off my cast by hand with giant plaster cutters and I was told I could use the sling at home when necessary. My left elbow was locked in the flexed position and wouldn't bend much. I went to Dr. Harry's office on the fourth floor of the Birks Building twice a week for treatment. At home, I was told to carry a gallon pail of water weighing ten pounds with my left hand for twenty minutes twice a day. I followed these instructions fervently; I wouldn't disappoint Dr. Harry!

The treatment at the office consisted of Dr. Harry putting his unshod heel in my left armpit and pulling on my forearm. I can remember hollering and trying to hold back tears. Dr. Harry persisted and always gave me twenty-five cents for hurting me. After four months, he had pulled my arm straight. My endurance awarded me four dollars, a vast sum for a ten-year-old kid in those Depression days.

When my dad offered to pay Dr. Harry for looking after my arm, he refused. Instead he said he might ask my dad for a few special favours. The first of many favours Dr. Harry asked of my dad was to fix the abscessed teeth of Harry's indigent patients. My dad's dental office was located at 321 Birks Building at 104 Street and Jasper Avenue, just a floor lower than Dr. Harry's.

After a few weeks Dad called a halt to Harry's request because the number of abscesses doubled each day and my dad's office was overrun with homeless people. Then Harry asked that on cold nights these same people be allowed to sleep on the floor in the dental office and use the office lavatory. Soon the Birks Building manager noted that the third floor toilets were a mess in the morning. The "super" of the building then had a talk with Dad, and Dr. Harry's request to "house the homeless" in Dad's office was stopped. This last episode strained their friendship slightly. Finally my dad wrote Dr. Harry a cheque to cover his professional fee for fixing my arm. Dad figured that paying him would be cheaper in the long run.

Over the years I would see a friendly Dr. Harry in the Birks Building. He always asked about my school work and if I was going to be a doctor. He seemed disappointed when he found out I was only interested in hockey, baseball and tennis.

I got to know him much better when I was eighteen. One summer night in 1947 I started vomiting and developed pain in the right side of my belly. Dr. Harry came to the house and diagnosed appendicitis and drove me in his car to the Mizz for surgery. Luckily his ancient Ford Model A Flivver made it across the High Level Bridge—unbeknownst to us, this would be its last trip. Once at the hospital, Dr. Harry arranged for Dr. Adamson to give me an anaesthetic—this time it was a spinal. Under anaesthetic Dr. Harry took my appendix out and I quickly recovered. Two days later he walked me to the streetcar stop on 109 Street where I caught the streetcar for home and he took the tram to his office in the Birks Building. Dr. Harry's Model A Ford had conked out completely. This time, my dad was glad to pay Dr. Weinlos' professional fee immediately—"with no sutures attached."

Dr. Harry and I became friends and we often met by chance, usually in the Birks Building. He always wanted to know what I planned to do when I graduated from high school. When I was twenty-one he was disappointed to learn that I had signed on as a Colonial Officer for three years and was to be stationed in Northern Nigeria. He tried to dissuade me and recommended I apply to medical school but my mind was made up and I sailed on the *Empress of Canada* in 1951 to Liverpool and then on the MV *Accra* to Lagos, Nigeria. Three years later, after being invalided home from Africa, having lost eighty pounds and recovering from Weil's disease, I realized that Dr. Harry was right and in 1954 I applied to medical school at the University of Alberta.

Dr. Harry always encouraged me during the preclinical years at med school when I would see him in the Birks Building. When I was a clinical clerk assigned to the Misericordia Hospital, he took over the teaching of my clinical rotation. Although he was a surgeon, Dr. Harry had patients on the pediatric and medical wards. He allowed me to do many deliveries, under his supervision, of his patients in the obstetrical unit. His surgical practice was huge and he had a varied group of general surgical patients as well as orthopedic, urological and plastic surgical cases. Dr. Harry was a whirlwind and many times we were making rounds at seven AM or midnight. He was one of the few doctors who looked after the Native people from the reserve in west Edmonton and Hobbema. Neither the colour of a person's skin or his race meant anything to him; everyone was treated with equal respect.

The nuns at the Misericordia Hospital loved him—he was their favourite doctor. He had the ability to get around their rules and religion and get his own way with the staff. Some of his poor patients at home were dehydrated and he used to beg the Mother Superior at the Mizz for IV fluids so he could give intravenous fluids to them in their own beds. The nuns always saw to it that he had free meals in the doctors' dining room and a place to sleep in the doctors' lounge; they even did his laundry and ironed the starched wing collars that he always wore. He was a bachelor and seldom went home.

When I interned at the Royal Alexandra Hospital in Edmonton Dr. Harry had many surgical patients on those wards as well. He always phoned me to help him with rounds even when I wasn't assigned to his surgical service. He was a fabulous teacher who related everything to the well-being of his patient. His reasoning was sound and he was knowledgeable and kind. I loved him.

One very cold night in February Dr. Harry phoned me to go on rounds with him at the "Alec." When I met him on the surgical floor after visiting hours his hands were red and cold-looking.

"Where are your gloves, Dr. Harry?"

"I gave them to one of my patients who didn't have any. I ran out of gas and had to walk to the hospital—all the way down Kingsway against that north wind. But I'm okay now. Apart from having cold hands I'm missing my supper."

"We better go to the hospital cafeteria and get you some supper now. You didn't run out of gas again, Dr. Harry?" I was calculating that he didn't have any money for supper or gas. I had just cashed my monthly hospital intern's cheque and had twenty dollars in my pocket.

"Here, Dr. Harry, I'll lend you five bucks for supper and gas. You can pay me back sometime."

"That should get me back to the Mizz after we have supper and do rounds. Thanks, Sterling."

It was the end of June when Harry repaid my loan. We met at Mary Samuels' house for a massive Jewish feast honouring Max Wershoff's appointment of Canadian ambassadorship to the UK and Dr. Harry's humanitarian way of practising medicine in Edmonton. My wife and I were invited because we were friends of Harry and my mother and dad were present because they were long-time friends of the Samuels'. I was also being honoured for having just passed my Liceniate of the Medical Council of Canada (LMCC), a national examination which allowed me to practise in Canada.

Supper was sumptuous but Dr. Harry was an hour late. I thought he might have run out of gas again and walked over from the Mizz. When he arrived all the guests had already finished the main entree. Harry bustled up to the table obviously famished and apologized for being late between mouthfuls.

"I'm so sorry to be late, Mary," said Dr. Harry. "The gefilte fish is marvelous but the soup a little cold..."

"What did you say, Dr. Harry? You are impossible. You arrive late at my dinner party and then complain that the soup is cold."

"I am so sorry, Mary, excuse my boorishness. Thank you very much for having me."

We had a rollicking evening, entertained by Dr. Harry's stories set on Ninety-seventh Street in Edmonton or at the Mizz. Max's eloquent tales of working in European embassies were also fascinating. As the evening closed, Mary Samuels told very funny Yiddish stories that her father had brought to Alberta from Europe. This was the last time I would see Dr. Harry but I have never forgotten him and his humanitarian ways.

Dr. Harry never sent out bills for all the work he did but he would mention his fee to patients once they were back at work. Patients paid their medical bills when they could. Edmontonians loved him for his kindness and altruism.

Medicine was in the Weinlos family blood both in Europe and Canada. Manuel, Harry's older brother, graduated from Vienna's medical school but sadly he was killed serving in the German Army Medical Corps in World War I. The remaining family came to Canada from Austria with their parents, Leah and Isaac, in 1921. The first five children were educated in Austria and the two youngest, Harry and Morris, were educated in Edmonton. Dr. Morris graduated from medicine at the U of A in 1929. Dr. Harry, the youngest brother, graduated a few years later. Harry and his brother Morris were among the first to enlist in the Canadian Medical Corp in September 1939. They both served in World War II until 1945 and were both discharged with the rank of major.

Dr. Morris recalled the following story about his brother, as quoted in the *Edmonton Journal* on August 27, 1977:

"Harry was hit in the head by a piece of German shrapnel during a Nazi bombing raid in Yorkshire. But he had the wound patched up quietly and never did report the incident. That was his attitude; he just didn't want to bother anyone."

Debby Shoctor, archivist for the Jewish Archives and Historical Society of Edmonton and Northern Alberta, sent me a copy of "a postcard from beyond" written by Dr. Harry, mailed in 1941 from England to Master Billy Lewchuk in Spirit River, Alberta.

This postcard, according to the archives, was delivered to Billy's sister in Spirit River, sixty-seven years late, in February 2008. Dr. Harry had treated Billy for a broken leg and other injuries at the Misericordia Hospital but was mobilized for the army overseas before Billy had recovered. Dr. Harry wrote these words of encouragement to Billy in his postcard: "Hope that when this card reaches you, you will be much healthier and stronger." Unfortunately Billy succumbed to his injuries. As reported in the *Edmonton Sun,* July 30, 1960, Dr. Weinlos did not find this out "until after the war, at which time he wrote a heartfelt letter of condolence to the Lewchuk family, which they still have."

In 1960 the *Edmonton Sun* reported that Dr. Harry made a house call to a rural farm. "The farmer was paralyzed by acute appendicitis but would not leave his abode because the plowing was not finished. Dr. Weinlos got on a pair of overalls and finished the plowing."

Dr. Harry provided free medical services to the O'Connell Institute, the Alberta Protestant Home, and the Good Shepherd Home for orphaned children; voluntary services to the Beulah Home for the Poor (which he helped to establish) and to orphaned children in the Atonement Home. He was active in the Edmonton Community Chest and provided voluntary services to the Home for Ex-Servicemen's Children.

Edmonton city fathers honoured Dr. Harry and his brother Dr. Morris by naming the Weinlos District of Edmonton and the Weinlos School after them. This primary school provides instruction for students with mild and moderate cognitive development. This is Edmonton's tribute to Dr. Morris Weinlos and to

Dr. Harry Weinlos, two outstanding city surgeons and teachers.

Dr. Harry was my doctor, mentor and friend for twenty years. His happy ways and compassion made him well-loved by me and his many patients in Northern Alberta.

ELIOT COHEN CORDAY, THE FAMOUS CARDIOLOGIST

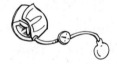

I first met Eliot Cohen when I was seven. It was during the Depression, in the spring of 1935, that Eliot's parents, Katie and David Cohen, asked our family—my mom, dad and my sister Shirley—to a Sunday dinner in Hay Lakes, Alberta. It was about noon on a hot day when we arrived at the Cohen store by car from Edmonton. The road east to Cooking Lake was gravel but from Cooking Lake on it was rutted and dusty. After thirty-one hard Canadian miles (fifty kilometres) we were dusty and irritable.

The Hay Lakes Mercantile sold a combination of grocery and dry goods, farm implements and hardware, and it had two ten-gallon gas pumps by the front door. The pumps were hand-operated and the gas flowed by gravity into the car, truck or tractor. They were located next to the horse trough filled with murky, alkali water. There were usually a few teams of horses hitched to the railing in front of the store. The store was open seven days a week. This Sunday afternoon, like most, farmers and church people had gathered at the store to shop, buy gas and gossip.

Dave was busy selling gas when we arrived. He gave us a welcome and then directed us to the upstairs living quarters where Katie was waiting for us. Dad and I parked and waited in line to gas up our old Ford Flivver. Mother and Shirley walked up the stairs of the store to the Cohen living quarters. Dave's three boys, Teddy, Eliot and Hy, were standing on the board-walk by the front door watching their father chew on his cigar stump and pump gas. Dave was a chunky short man who wore bib GWG red-strap overalls. That day his greasy denims were soaked with gas and when he attempted to light a large Eddy match on the seat of his pants there was a little explosion. Before he could light his cigar stump, Dave was engulfed in flames.

Dad dashed out of our car. The three sons and Dad each grabbed one of Dave's limbs and threw him in the horse trough. No one was hurt and Dave sheepishly declared that he was "okay" and then went into the store to change his wet clothes. This episode put a bit of a damper on Dave's mercurial temper and he seemed subdued. Eliot, a medical student at the University of Alberta, tended his father's minor burns to his hands and then we all gathered in the dining room above the store for a delicious Jewish meal. The meal included borsht with lokshen and gefilte fish and mounds of shredded cheese, matzos and whipping cream. There was honey and figs for dessert and the men drank homemade wine.

I got to know Eliot much better four years later, during the spring of 1939. Eliot was in his final year of medicine at the U of A when the Dean of Medicine, Johnny Ower, declared that unless Eliot passed his pre-med Latin exam he would not graduate with the rest of the medical class. My mother, Elizabeth, was a Latin scholar, so three times a week Eliot arrived at our house for Latin lessons and to have his homework corrected by my mother. His Latin homework was always done and he arrived on time; he was polite and friendly. He had a very rigorous schedule at medical school but he always had time for me and we talked about the practice of medicine and about his family as well as mine.

Eliot was a handsome slim man. His suits were always smart and well-pressed and his black hair was combed back. He had a pencil-thin black moustache and was always well groomed whenever we met.

Eliot's academic record was always superlative except for Latin. At the U of A he started his studies in electrical engineering but later on he switched to the Faculty of Medicine. Eliot, after studying with my mother, passed the Latin exam with flying colours and graduated from the University of Alberta Faculty of Medicine in 1940. After graduation, Eliot married his sweetheart, Marion, in Edmonton. Then he joined the RCAF where he served as a Canadian Air Force doctor in World War II.

In 1945, Eliot and Marion moved to New York City to be with Eliot's brother, Ted Corday. It was in NYC that Eliot and Marion changed their name to Corday as well. Some anti-Jewish racism had developed in Canada and the USA in the 1930s and Teddy had felt this underlying racism. When he started to write, produce and direct for the stage and radio in NYC he was the first in the family to change his name to Corday. After the name change, Ted worked with NBC. When Eliot arrived, Ted was established in theatre and radio. They both looked Spanish or perhaps French Canadian and so the French name of Corday fit.

Eliot started a medical residency in NYC in cardiology and trained with Dickenson Richards, a Nobel Prize winner in medicine. Richards and Corday, with Dr. Arthur Masters, refined the early Masters Two-Step Stair Test. Eliot, with his engineering experience, developed the modern cardiac stress testing and EKG monitoring performed when walking on a treadmill. Again with Dr. Richards, Eliot developed research studies that led to the development of cardiac catheterization. Eliot was only thirty-two years old at the time.

In 1949, Eliot and Marion moved to Los Angeles and worked in the Cedars of Lebanon Hospital where he developed radio-isotope studies that became the forerunner of modern nuclear cardiology. Soon he was the leading cardiologist in the USA and contributed to four new fields: stress testing, ambulatory EKG monitoring, cardiac catheterization and nuclear cardiology.

Eliot was not only a researcher and teacher but a dedicated physician. He was the cardiologist who looked after William Randolph Hearst and President Dwight Eisenhower when he was in the White House. He was chief consulting cardiologist for the United States Army and looked after many of its soldiers including five-star General Omar Bradley, who was supreme commander of the US Army in the 1940s. Busy as he was, he also looked after my aging Aunt Iva when she lived in Los Angeles.

When my Aunt Iva phoned Eliot's office for an appointment the receptionist told her that "Dr. Corday is not accepting new patients."

Iva said, "I'm a long-time friend of Eliot's family. Would you please tell him Iva Haynes of Edmonton and Hay Lakes, Alberta, phoned. I'll leave my number and perhaps Dr. Corday could call me."

Eliot called the next day and spoke about the Haynes family with fondness and his Latin tutoring in 1939 by my mother. He said he would be "delighted to see Iva about any cardiac problems at any time."

The receptionist gave Iva an appointment.

Aunt Iva developed atrial fibrillation that was resistant to treatment. Eliot spent time with Iva and diagnosed a toxic goiter and thyrotoxicosis. Once the thyroid problem was treated by a thyroidectomy, her atrial fibrillation was relatively easy to control.

Iva's condition greatly improved and she always raved about the great care she had received from the famous Canadian cardiologist, Dr. Eliot Corday.

In the 1960s Eliot was elected president of the American College of Cardiology. He and his close friend, cardiac surgeon Michael DeBakey, advocated federal funding for cardiovascular research. As a professor at UCLA he was involved with teaching the latest cardiac diagnostic and treatment methods internationally. He also organized live TV interchanges with physicians globally including those behind the Iron Curtain. As the David Cohen family had emigrated from Lithuania to Canada in 1901, I am sure Eliot was aware of his Jewish family ties in Lithuania and Russia.

President Ronald Reagan honoured Eliot Corday with this letter:

> Sharing your knowledge and skills with physicians of other countries, you have served as an Ambassador of Goodwill. Your efforts dramatically demonstrate that America stands ready to work with others to help solve common problems.

Eliot Corday was born in Prince Rupert, British Columbia, in 1913. He was raised and educated in Alberta, British Columbia and the USA and died in Los Angeles on February 10, 1999. He was a humble man who gave of himself, never forgot a friend and asked nothing in return.

TATTOOS AND TB

Cecelia was a sixteen-year-old Inuit woman with tattoos and TB. On September 6, 1957, she flew from Tuk-Tuk, Northwest Territories, to Edmonton, Alberta, to be treated for TB of the spine at the Charles Camsell Indian Hospital. Cecelia had massive tuberculosis lymph node swellings in each groin. As a medical student in my first semester of third year at the Univeristy of Alberta, I was assigned to look after Cecelia. My first thought was that she was an interesting case. After a time, I found Cecelia was also a dear: she was kind, humble and very lonely. I kept seeing her for the greater part of my academic year. I wrote a complete history and physical of many of her medical problems and kept up with my progress notes. You might say Cecelia was my baby. She was an attractive, rotund young woman with a deeply tattooed face and inner thighs. The orthopedic department doctors saw Cecelia in consultation when she arrived and they recommended that she be placed in a full body cast and have needle biopsies and aspiration of her chronic psoas tubercular abscesses in each groin. Tests came back positive for tubercle bacillus and the biopsy of the lymph node showed caseation necrosis and confirmed TB. I was delighted that my aspiration and biopsies were positive, a professional first, though I felt sorry for Cecelia. She was not thrilled with the results.

I was asked by the orthopedic surgeon to apply the body cast with the help of the orderly in the cast room and Mario, the pediatric resident. The orthopedic wing of the hospital had two large wards side by side, one for men and the other for women.

After a few months, Cecelia started complaining that the body cast was too tight. Every few weeks I would have to cut her cast and the orderly and I would reapply a new one.

"Cecelia," I said, "why do you think the cast seems to be getting tighter?"

"I don't know. Maybe because the food is really good here and I don't get much exercise. But lately when I eat too much I get a sick feeling, like I want to puke. Guess I'll have to cut down on my eats. Willie, my friend in the next ward, says I should go on a diet. I guess you knew Willie and I are from the same village?"

"I'll ask the dietician to put you on diet. Maybe I should talk to Willie and see what he thinks?"

"Oh, Doc, I wouldn't do that. His English ain't too good."

"Okay, Cecelia, if that's what you want. By the way, I've often wondered why you have blue-black tattoos on your face and inner thighs. Are they religious tribal marks?"

The circles radiated out from her nose. The black lines looked like they had been drawn with a compass, the point centred on the tip of her nose.

"Yes, Doc, you got it. My aunt was the spirit doc for my tribe. She tattooed me with lamp black and later with charcoal scraped from the bottom of our copper kettle—that's what made the ones on my chin and cheeks. Auntie took bone needles and coated the sinew thread with blackened seal oil. Like a seamstress, she sewed those tattoos onto my face and legs. Sometimes they use black gunpowder. They's all permanent, don't wash off. Our men like that kinda stuff too. Tattoos help them sight in their guns, so the men say. My people have been doing tattoos for hundreds of years."

"What do the tattoos mean?"

"Well, Doc, the circles are my charms—they make me have good babies. The small circles on each side of my mouth show walrus tusks. They protect me from bad men and bears. The tattoos on my thighs were done when I was twelve years old. They'll give me an easy labour when I have my baby. They are my medicine tattoos."

"Should I change your cast sometime?"

"Yeah, Doc, I sure would like you to change it. Could you do it today?"

"Not today but maybe at the end of the week. I'll have to check with Mario, the chief pediatric resident. He's in charge of all the kids."

"I ain't a child, Doc, I'm a woman."

"Okay Cec. I'll try and do it on Friday."

On Friday the orderly and I bi-valved the body cast. When we rolled Cecelia out of the cast the nurse gave her a bath and we all noticed she had a marked striae and swelling of her lower abdomen. Was it an ovarian tumour—a dermoid or massive serous cystadenoma? I called Mario, the chief resident and I suggested that I get x-rays of her abdomen. Mario told me before I did anything to please get a pregnancy test and take it from there.

I was sure that Cecelia had not been pregnant when she

arrived but I wondered how in the world she could have had sex in a body cast. Making love must have been difficult. And who could possibly be the father? The man must have been a contortionist, a wiry magician or both.

At that time I had two choices in ordering a biological pregnancy test—a "frog test" or a "rabbit test." The rabbit test consisted of injecting a sample of the tested woman's urine into an immature female rabbit. The rabbit was then sacrificed and a post mortem performed to examine the bunny's ovaries. If the woman was pregnant, the rabbit's ovaries would have changed in response to the presence of the hormone human chorionic gonadotropin (hCG) only secreted by pregnant women. In the frog test (also called a Bufo Test) a woman's urine was injected into an amphibian and if the urine contained hCG, within twenty-four hours the frog would lay eggs. I thought the rabbit test was more appropriate. It came back positive for pregnancy.

Over the next six months I dutifully changed the cast and did my prenatal assessments while her fetus got bigger and bigger. Cecelia never would tell me who the father was although I suspected it was Willie, the lithe eighteen-year-old Inuit man from the next ward.

Cecelia delivered a big baby boy in the Misericordia Hospital maternity ward, without the body cast and without any difficulty. She knew it would be easy. She said afterwards, "My tattoos sure helped me through labour."

When I put the baby to her breast to suckle, Cecelia thanked us all.

"I'm gonna name the baby after you, Doc—William. But we're going to call him Willie for short."

I thanked Cecelia for remembering that my first name was William. But I'm still not sure who the child was really named after, me or the other Willie in the adjacent orthopedic wing.

Six months of treatment at the Charles Camsell Hospital in Edmonton led to the recovery of both Cecelia and her friend Willie. They were declared "cured of TB" and returned to the Arctic and their community with their happy baby boy, William. He was a joyful addition to their extended Inuit family.

THE JOLLY GREEN GIANT

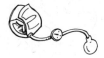

My first week on duty as a junior intern at the Royal Alexan-dra Hospital in Edmonton was most unusual. When I had graduated two months earlier from the University of Alberta in medicine, I was broke. The only well-paying job open to me for the two months before my internship began on July 1 was work-ing for the city Sewer and Water Department.

When I arrived at the hospital to start my internship, after two months of hard manual labour, I was outfitted with three white uniforms and I bought a pair of expensive, comfortable white buck shoes and white shoe polish. But my new white ap-pearance didn't address my face and arms, which were tanned, my callused fingers and palms and my broken fingernails. My grimy hands belied my academic background in medicine.

My first duty was to start an IV with a cannula in the arm of a sweet, white-haired woman. Her veins, when touched, rolled under her fragile skin. My rough, huge hands were callused but with the help of the nurse I managed to start the IV by threading a catheter up her vein.

When I got the IV running, this elderly patient asked me, "What kind of work did you do before you became a doctor? You seem a happy sort but your broken nails scratched my skin."

"I'm so sorry, Ma'am, it was unintentional."

I explained that I'd just finished working for the Edmonton Sewer and Water Department, a job I had taken to make enough money to help last my pregnant wife and me through the year. My intern's wages were only twenty dollars a month, I told her. I apologized again for the rough state of my hands and ragged nails.

I then reported to the surgical ward, which was where things became interesting for a very green junior house doctor on his first night on-call.

After midnight I was called to attend to a surgical patient on Three South that had just died from advanced carcinomatosis. I phoned the attending doctor, contacted the priest on duty and talked to the relatives.

Then the "probey" (a young RN in training) said, "Come quickly, Doctor, the dead man just moved."

I rushed back to the two-bed ward and found that the movement was due to early rigor mortis. "Whew," I said, followed by a four-letter word!

The night was not over. I returned to my basement room in the 1908 isolation hospital where the interns' quarters were located. I had just fallen asleep when the nurse on Third Surgical phoned again about a man in the private room who had just had a gastrectomy.

"You better come up fast," said the charge nurse. "The patient has just had gastric surgery by Dr. Richards. Don't fall asleep on me, Doctor, I need you here stat."

As I entered the ward I saw a pale, sweaty, middle-aged

man. I noted a musty smell in the room. His heart rate was 150 beats per minute and his temperature 104 degrees Fahrenheit. His blood pressure was dropping rapidly and he was short of breath. His wound felt bubbly. I remembered the words "subcutaneous emphysema" from my fourth-year surgical lectures. The skin of his abdomen was blistered. The musty smell of old hay was overwhelming at the bedside. I realized that the patient had gas gangrene.

"Nurse," I said, "this man has gas gangrene. Speed up the intravenous and I'll thread an IV plastic catheter up the vein of his left ankle. Please call the lab to take cultures and do a complete blood count."

"Sorry, Doctor, all the lab work after midnight has to be by the intern. That's you. I'll get the cut-down tray right away."

"Me? I don't even know where the lab is."

"You'll have to find out, Doctor."

"I'll take the cultures first and do a gram stain on the blister fluid and later the complete blood count." Then I added, "I'll phone Dr. Hal Richards, the attending surgeon, right away."

"Are you sure about this diagnosis, Doctor? I've been nursing for twenty-five years and have never seen a case."

"Yes, I'm positive. Please get the culture swabs and the blood culture bottles. We'll need to give large doses of aqueous penicillin intravenously by a rapid push. He'll need more surgery."

"Are you certain, Doctor? Isn't this your first week on duty. You may have to do the blood crossmatch yourself."

"Are you sure I have to do the crossmatching? Now I'll have to get Dr. Richards to come immediately. This patient will need more surgery."

"You know what Dr. Richards is like after midnight."

"Are you with me or not, Nurse? This man is in bad shape. This is a real emergency, just like you said. I'll call the attending surgeon right now."

Dr. Richards came immediately and approved of my treatment and agreed with my diagnosis. He then made arrangements to take the patient back to the operating room for complete debridement of his wound. Luckily, he asked me to help him and ordered the medical technologist to come in to do the lab work and the blood crossmatch. I was relieved. We worked all night in the OR but the patient died at dawn of septic shock.

For the rest of my two months on the surgical service the nurses deferred to me. They liked the big, tanned, happy doctor with rough, callused hands.

One probey said, "He's a happy enough guy although he looks like a farmer. But the chief of surgery, Dr. Richards, actually likes him. Seems sort of funny, because Dr. Richards usually eats interns alive."

In my green surgical "scrub suit" uniform I had achieved notoriety. The staff throughout the hospital called me "the jolly green giant" and my nickname stuck for the rest of the year.

WHITE BOY

Almost fifty years ago, I left the Royal Alexandra Hospital interns' quarters in the basement of the old infectious disease building in Edmonton, Alberta. I had taken a residency in general practice at the Kaiser Permanente Foundation Hospital in Oakland, California. Having passed the American Medical Association's long and difficult licensing examinations, I was looking forward to making three hundred and fifty dollars (US) per month as a medical resident. Dr. Martin Shearn, who was in charge of education at this large teaching hospital, promised me that the administration would do their utmost to give me extra work. I would be well paid at twenty dollars per hour as an ER Doc or a house-call Doc during my nights off.

My first night as a house-call Doc was a difficult one. It started in an elegant Berkeley Hills bathroom where I packed a wealthy lawyer's nose because of a nosebleed. I instructed him "not to take Aspirin or warfarin blood thinners" and to go to the Permanente Clinic the next day. After his nose stopped bleeding I received an emergency call from my dispatcher telling me to go to Richmond to see a woman who was vomiting and had abdominal pain. I had no time to go home and change my blood-stained white shirt and pants.

Before the dispatcher hung up, she said, "You might want to go first to a Richmond City Police Precinct and have a cop go with you to make the call; the man on the phone sounded southern and swore a lot." The apartment was in the black section on the fourth floor of a brownstone walkup, she told me.

"I'm okay, I won't need a cop."

"It's your funeral," she said. "You'll know the place. The apartment is above a bar with a big red sign in the window promoting Schlitz Beer—can't miss it. The street lights are dim in those black districts, but watch for the sign."

With second thoughts about asking a cop to accompany me, I got into my yellow VW beetle and headed for the City of Richmond, a map of the Bay Area on my lap.

The buldings in the area were dirty and brown in the "colored section" and the Schlitz Beer sign cast a ruby-like glow on the building and the correct address.

I parked by the bar, picked up my doctor's bag and got out of my car, locking it behind me. Suddenly about six large young African American men surrounded me. The bar had just closed and in the darkness I could only see teeth and eyes and large shapes.

Their leader said, "What are you doin' here, white boy?"

I waved my doctor's bag and said, "I was called, the patient's son told us that his mother was sick on the fourth floor."

Just then I heard a shout from the upper balcony. "You damned bums leave the Doc alone. You touch him and I'll whip your asses, ya'll hear. I'll be right down jist as soon as I gets my Saturday night special loaded."

In about three minutes a huge man appeared beside my car in a white T-shirt and shorts. A .38 was jammed into the waistband of his jockey shorts.

"Thanks for comin', ya doin' all right? My ma, she's from Louisiana, by Lake Charles there. She been sick for about three or four days. Upchuckin' and moaning with pain. She cain't shit none—not even fart. Ma's been with me here for almost a year. Took her to that local Doc for the past two days. He's close, around the corner, but he don't do her any good. I'll take your bag, Doc, and show ya the way; it's three stories up. My name's Jethro—gimme your hand, Doc."

"Good to meet you, Jethro. I'll follow behind."

As we walked up the stairs, Jethro told me that he was a stevedore for Kaiser Aluminum and made good money working on the docks in Oakland. He assured me that he had good Kaiser Permanent Health Insurance.

When I entered the three-room apartment, I could smell feces coming from the largest bedroom.

"Come on in here, Doc. The wife and some of the kids are in here with Ma."

I was flabbergasted as we entered the dimly lit bedroom. There was a wash basin full of fecal vomit and beside the white-haired woman were four little kids and a strikingly beautiful woman. Jethro's wife was washing the ill woman. It looked like the four kids and the sick older woman shared the same bed.

"Hi, Mrs. Jethro, your mother-in-law looks sick."

"Yes, she is a sick old woman and has been for four or five days. I kept asking Jethro to phone Kaiser Permanente Hospital and get her proper care. Jethro's stubborn and didn't want to carry her in—he wanted a house call for Mother Mary."

Mother Mary was markedly dehydrated. Her eyes were

sunken, lips dry and her skin hung on her bones. Her abdomen was distended and she had hyperactive bowel sounds. The kids were silent and scared-looking in the poor light.

"Don't mash me none, Doc, I's too sick. Jist let me die," she moaned.

"Jethro, please get me a good light—your mother looks terrible."

"What do you think, Doc? Mom is a good, honest God-fearing woman. Her parents were slaves in Mississippi but she educated herself in Louisiana. Ma can read and write some."

"Jethro, we'll have to get the ambulance. Your mother has a bowel obstruction, probably a piece of rotten bowel, and is vomiting up feces. She has an infection from the bowel and has no fluid left in her—she's like a prune."

"I thought her upchucking smelt like shit. She shore do look dry, as you say."

"Where's your phone? I'll call the Permanente Ambulance Service; if I call, you won't have to pay for the ambulance."

"Geez, thanks, Doc. The phone's in the kitchen."

About an hour later we all arrived at the MacArthur Street ambulance entrance. The medics carried Mother Mary into the emergency room where I could examine her under a decent light. "Shore do 'preciate all this here attention. Does you think I'm a goner? Never been in a hospital before or looked after by a whitey Doc."

"You're pretty sick, Mary, but we're going to do some x-rays and take some blood out of your arm. Then we'll run some sugar and salt into your veins. Dr. Angus McLeod, a surgeon, is going to see you. You'll definitely have to have surgery in an hour or so. Dr. McLeod will do the surgery. He talks kinda funny, he's from Scotland. He's a bit matter-of-fact but he means well and he's good. Trust him, Mary. The nurse anaesthetist will put you to sleep soon and you'll wake up on the surgical ward."

"I gotta trust him and the Lord too, Doc. Gotta look after those four grandkids, the youngest she's jist knee high. She's named Mary after me."

Mother Mary had a mechanical small bowel obstruction and a loop of gangrenous ileum. The surgery and resection went well and she was back in the ward before dawn.

Jethro and I had breakfast in the hospital cafeteria and were at Mary's side when she returned from the surgical theatre.

I saw Mary every day with Jethro until she was discharged ten days later. Mary, Jethro and I occasionally had lunch together at the hospital over the next two months.

When I left to return to Canada, Mother Mary and her family continued to send me cards of remembrance at Christmas and Easter. I had been adopted as their "white boy" doctor.

The Old Burn Unit

The smell of burnt flesh, coliform and pseudomonas infections was overpowering when entering the old burn unit at the Vancouver General Hospital (VGH) on Twelfth Avenue in the 1960s. The burn unit, about fifty years old, could house over 150 adult patients, mostly firemen.

As a surgical resident living in the residents' quarters a block away I was always available. During the few months of my residency, I was privileged to work as an assistant with three plastic surgeons and burn specialists—Drs. Bob Cowan, Douglas Courtemache and occasionally Robert Langston, who initially set up the burn unit in British Columbia. They were an exceptional group of men and with the help of the concerned, efficient nurses we ran the burn unit.

They subscribed to this doctrine:
"Those who the heights attained and kept
Did not achieve by sudden flight
But they whilst their companions slept
Climbed slowly upward in the night."

These three surgeons were dedicated and shunned the easy money to be made by doing facelifts, boobs and tubes, tummy tucks and other cosmetic surgery. Burned men and women always came first.

During the week, I was assigned to place firemen—some with 80 percent body burn—into baths of warm water called Hubbard tanks. I debrided their wounds while I gave them intermittent doses of morphine. The stench was always present but the firemen often cracked jokes while I cut burnt flesh away with sharp scissors and scalpel. I never heard a single complaint. On Saturdays I helped the plastic surgeons with multiple skin grafting.

There was one particular man whom I remember. Joe was a stoic, tough young man who had been employed as a linesman for BC Hydro. After a bad storm he was clearing downed lines at the top of a cedar pole when he was electrocuted by thousands of volts. His hand went into tetany and he clutched the hot wire and then fell from the pole and broke his right femur. Luckily the wire was jerked from his grasp during the fall.

The wound of entry was his right hand; the massive exit wound was his right foot. The tissue damage to his right chest wall was severe and he was transferred from the emergency room of the Okanagan Hospital to VGH. Dr. Bob Cowan was the attending doctor. Initially, Dr. Cowan treated Joe for burn shock and completed fasciotomies to the right leg. Later, an orthopedic surgeon stabilized the right femur by inserting an intermedullary rod.

Some of the right ribs were badly burnt and the necrotic bone was completely removed by Dr. Cowan, leaving Joe with an unstable right chest wall covered by skin and pleura. Joe managed, even as the balloon-like soft tissue covering of the right chest wall went in and out with each breath. The gangrene of his right foot resulted in partial amputation of his forefoot. Joe slowly went into renal failure. Renal dialysis was not available in BC at this time but Dr. Cowan successfully treated him with peritoneal dialysis.

Eventually, Joe was discharged from the burn hospital and went back to the Okanagan where he ran a gas station, towing service, and rural grocery and liquor store. Joe was an uncomplaining, likeable, very busy man who, years later, spoke fondly of "his doc," Bob Cowan.

I was glad to hear that the new VGH burn unit, the British Columbia Professional Fire Fighters Burn and Plastic Surgery Unit, became available this century. The burned men and women of BC and the Yukon deserve it.

CARIBOO

Bear Facts

When I practised medicine forty-five years ago in the frontier town of Williams Lake, in the Cariboo region of British Columbia, bear attacks were not uncommon. There is an old adage that says, "If it's black go back, if there's a hump be a lump." The two situations that I was involved with were grizzly attacks when there was no time to be "a lump."

The first case was that of a laconic rancher, formerly a marine then professional hockey player in the West Coast Hockey League for the Seattle team. Johnny Mac was physically tough and ran a stump cattle ranch in the foothills of the Ulgatcho Mountains when his hockey days were over. Sometimes, he worked as a guide or faller for the P&T logging outfit. His neighbours called him Ulgatcho Johnny. He was a bear of a man.

One spring day Johnny was cutting firewood with a commercial chainsaw and a double bitted axe. He was about a mile from his log house under the canopy of a West Coast cedar when he was surprised by a small sow grizzly bear. The bear immediately attacked. Johnny's chainsaw was idling and his axe was leaned against the tree. There was no time to run or climb.

When I saw him in the Cariboo Memorial Hospital, Johnny—normally a man of few words—told me the whole story. "You know, Doc, I just cut part of her front paw off when she reared up. Then I backhanded her shoulder to the bone and jammed my saw. She was bleeding bad but kept coming. She tore off my right boot and crunched my leg bad. She cuffed me across the arm and got my face. Then I got my two-headed axe and gave her a good one in the snout. She run off spraying the March corn snow with red blood."

"What happened next, Johnny?"

"Well, Doc, I tore the sleeves out of my wool shirt and got a good tight dressing on. Stopped the bleeding and all. Hobbled up to my pickup and drove home. My good wife took over then. The rest is history and here I am in Willie's Puddle."

His wife tended his wounds then drove him to their closest neighbours where he was taken to the Alexis Creek Red Cross Hospital. The nurse gave IVs and morphine and he was transported to the old grey clapboard Williams Lake hospital. Barney Ringwood, a local surgeon, treated his many wounds under ether anaesthesia. I gave him blood transfusions. The lacerated tendons were marked with silk suture for future reference and repair. The massive wounds were closed over rubber drains. Large doses of aqueous penicillin and streptomycin were given. Johnny was transferred the next day to the Vancouver General Hospital. The next morning, Johnny's neighbours tracked the grizzly by the blood trail on the snow. They found her dead. She had managed to run about a mile before she bled to death.

When the September hunting season rolled around in the Ulgatcho Mountains, Johnny had horses in his corral and his tack ready. He had recovered from the surgery and was leading another series of hunts for moose, deer, mountain goat and sheep. He was an excellent guide and was booked up by American hunters for the entire fall. For the first time, Johnny decided that this year there would be no bear hunt. He had reached his "limit" for grizzlies.

The second encounter was with my hunting buddies, Jack and Bob, and our Native guides, Baptiste Dester and Scotty Greg. We had ridden from Dester's ranch in the Tatla Lake region to Wheeler's Bottom. We followed the course of the Klinaklini River to the base of Pike's Peak in the Coast Range Mountains. It was a tough ride and we had to swim the horses across the ford before the country opened up into Wheeler's Bottom. We were hunting deer, moose and Rocky Mountain goats.

We set our tents close to the river and hobbled our horses in the pasture. As we cooked supper on a campfire we heard what sounded like another horse galloping down the trail. It was moving fast and as it approached us in the twilight we could tell it wasn't a horse but it seemed the size of a pony. In the shooting flames of our fire we could see it was a large bear with a hump. A grizzly. It ran past in a flash and was gone.

The next day we each shot a moose. Bob shot a dry cow, I got a yearling and at twilight Jack shot a bull moose. As the light was fading, Jack decided to gut the animal and prop the abdominal cavity open and then retrieve the animal with packhorses the next morning. The moose lay among willows and poplars on a high hummock. Jack blazed the trees close by and marked the spot in the bottomland, then he headed to camp for supper.

The next morning at dawn Jack left to locate his moose. Bob and I retrieved the three packhorses we would need to pack Jack's moose out. We had aptly named the nags Knothead One, Knothead Two and Knothead Three because they all tried to rub their loads off their backs. We placed the packsaddles on their backs, tightened the cinches and put bridles on them. Finally we followed the trail to the blazed trees. After about twenty minutes, we heard a shot close by. Knothead Three was really spooked and ran back to the pasture. The other two were in frenzy but we managed to hold them and quiet them down before we walked into the willow and poplar forest.

Bob and I were walking into the willow marsh when we spotted Jack sitting on a dry hummock about one hundred yards (ninety metres) away holding his bleeding foot in the air. There was no sign of the moose.

"What happened?" we shouted.

"That big grizzly was after my gutted moose. He came at me like an express train. I got one shot in, missed and dropped my rifle. Then I climbed this poplar as high as I could go. The bear tried to drag me out of the tree. Tore my laced boot from my right foot and clawed my foot and leg. He must have heard your horses coming and took off, thank God. My foot looks kind of bad, Doc."

I examined the foot. "Looks like he tore out the extensor tendons of your toes and slashed the muscles of your leg. We'll get a dressing on this and get you back to camp. We'll use my white T-shirt for a dressing, just put it on clean this morning. You can ride Knothead Number One back to camp."

"Where is your moose?" asked Bob.

"That SOB grizzly dragged that thousand-pound moose carcass about a hundred yards. He was feeding on it when I came into the open part here. He must have been super strong to have dragged it so far."

"We'll get Scottie and Baptiste to pack your moose out while we have a good look at your foot in camp. Let's get you up on this horse."

It was a slow trip back to camp. Once there, I boiled gallons of river water on the Coleman stove and washed out Jack's lacerated foot with soap and boiled water. I gave him a couple of Frosst 292s and four sulfa tablets from my medicine kit. I ground up some more sulfa tablets between two spoons and sprinkled the powder over the wound. After about two hours of debriding the laceration with a new razor blade, I put on a large dressing of T-shirts and an elastic bandage. The other men broke camp and loaded the pack animals for the emergency eight-hour trip back to Baptiste's ranch.

I rode with Jack and held his foot up when we had to ford the Klinaklini River on the way back. With a Chevy pickup full of moose and one stoic patient we headed for "The Lake," stopping for a change of dressing and a shot of morphine at the Alexis Creek Red Cross Hospital. At midnight we got Jack into the War Memorial Hospital where I immediately changed the dressings and gave IV morphine, penicillin and streptomycin. Margie, the hospital cook, cooked us a huge supper of moose T-bone steaks in the wee hours of the morning. The one thousand pounds of bull moose meat proved to be even tougher than Jack's personality.

The next morning Jack was still in pain and the foot and tendons were already infected and swollen. He was transferred to the large Royal Columbian Hospital in New Westminster where he recovered under the care of Dr. Billy Graham, a Royal Columbian plastic surgeon.

THE ALEXIS CREEK RED CROSS OUTPOST HOSPITAL

In 1960 Dr. Barney Ringwood, a surgeon from Williams Lake, BC, was mooching around the attic of the Alexis Creek Red Cross Hospital when he made two notable finds. The first was a saddlebag, which he found under the eaves of the roof. In the saddlebag was a set of surgical instruments. There were bone saws, hemostats, needle drivers, needles, scalpels and a prolific collection of metal catheters wrapped in velvet. They looked new but had probably been there for forty years. The second find, discovered in the attic, was a portable rectangular box containing a cathode tube; it was lined with velvet and it too looked pristine. On the side was a large silver crank handle. Accompanying this primitive x-ray unit was a bulky cassette and film impregnated with silver salts.

When Dr. Ringwood showed the second find to the four doctors of the War Memorial Hospital in "The Lake," we gathered around this interesting relic and tried it out using modern x-ray cassettes and films. We took x-rays of hands and arms while cranking the handle vigorously and initiating a visible spark from the cathode tube. The developed films were hazy but I'm sure they would would have been useful in taking post reduction x-rays of new fractures. Dr. Ringwood sent both these items to the BC Medical Museum in Vancouver.

As I was at one time an attending physician at the Alexis Creek Hospital, Dr. Ringwood's finds sparked my interest in early frontier medical care, the hospital and the men and women who dedicated their lives to the care of the ill.

The first log hospital in the Chilcotin region was built on Alex Graham's land in Alexis Creek in 1912. The site was on a hill overlooking Highway 20. Highway 20 was a terrible road and for years there was a warning sign posted close to Alexis Creek that read "This Road Is Impassable, Not Even Jackass-able." Eighty years ago it must have been nothing more than a cow trail, and driving or riding to and from the hospital must have been an arduous job.

The first resident physician and midwife was Dr. William Wright, an Australian. Prior to coming to Alexis Creek he had been a ship's doctor who sailed the South China seas. His last medical practice began in 1912 and ended with his death in Vancouver in 1924. The first baby born in the hospital was Bill Graham in 1915; many babies have been born there since.

Doc Wright's companion and able assistant was nurse Mary Goode, who was also Australian. Late at night the Doc was prone to say, while giving advice, "Well, why don't you put a little iodine on it." Then Mary would take over and institute a plan of treatment and mollify the patient.

A small cozy lean-to was built for the two and attached to the hospital. I'm sure it was a welcome beacon on the long winter nights in the chilly Chilcotin. In a painting by Dr. Wright, held at the Williams Lake Museum Archives, the hospital and staff quarters are easily seen against the snowbound property.

Dr. Wright travelled the Chilcotin and the Cariboo region by saddle horse, buggy and cutter. In her book *History and Happenings in the Chilcotin*, Irene Stangoe relates Mike Farwell's description of driving Dr. Wright from the Beecher House Hotel at Riske Creek to the Farwell home at the Pothole Ranch to attend Mrs. Farwell.

"The good doctor, who had been celebrating his birthday, not too wisely, was asleep in the sleigh when Mike started his descent to the river down a hog's back with a steep gully on each side called the 'the toboggan slide.' It was just wide enough for the sleigh. Farwell wakened and warned the Doc, 'Hang on tight because if you go overboard here, you'll break your neck for sure.' The horses had gone two steps when Doc took a nosedive over the front of the sleigh, taking Farwell with him. The team stopped dead. In the melee, 'the back of the sleigh tipped up and under the seat an open tin of cigarettes sprayed over us like confetti at a wedding. I got out of the mess immediately but the Doc was lying under the tongue of the sleigh, between the horses, on his face and dead to the world.'

"Mike wrestled the big man from the brink of the bank and dumped him, like a sack of potatoes, into the back of the sleigh and continued onto the Pothole Ranch [now part of the Gang Ranch].

"The next day Doc Wright commented, 'It's a most curious thing; I've had a complete lapse of memory since the morning at the hotel.'"

There have been many eccentric and able physicians in Alexis Creek. In 1938 an English surgeon, Dr. Hallows, came with two nurses, Nan Hopkins and Ruby Craig. During this time, Lord Nuffield of England donated an iron lung to the Alexis Creek Hospital. Lord Nuffield hadn't realized that the town of Alexis

Creek had no electricity, so the iron lung sat in its massive crate unopened. For years this machine sat by the entrance inside the hospital where it became a fixture in the corner. After a few years it became a repository for scarves, toques, sweaters, galoshes, cowboy boots and even one large pair of red winter underwear (never used). In 1945, Dr. Sallows uncovered the machine and had it shipped to the Vancouver General Hospital. It was put to good use by paralyzed patients in the polio epidemics of the late 1940s and early '50s.

The provincial government paid a stipend of twelve hundred dollars per year to keep the hospital open until it was taken over by the Red Cross; it was renamed the Alexis Creek Red Cross Hospital in 1949.

As time passed and living conditions improved in this remote area, this two-ward hospital installed central heating. An English nurse practitioner, Lillian Whitesides (otherwise known as "old Whitesides"), staffed it. The hospital served about fifteen hundred people including the Native people from as far away as the Anahim Lake reserve, a distance of about 130 miles (about 210 kilometres).

Public health nurses and the Gray Nun nurse Sister Roberte did yeoman service in the backwoods country as visiting practitioners. Sister Roberte was a competent and dedicated nurse and an excellent diagnostician. I can remember her bringing in twelve Indian babies with meningitis during a blizzard in January 1962. They stayed in the Cariboo Memorial Hospital and they all recovered in ten days but it was months before their families came to town to pick up their kids. They all survived thanks to the quick action of Sister Roberte. I asked her why she chose such an isolated job. She said she liked lonesome places and the job satisfied her calling as a nurse. After fifteen years the Catholic Church recalled Sister Roberte from the Chilcotin, saying that she had lost contact with her God, and sent her to a cloistered retreat in Montreal. I never saw my friend again.

In 1979 an ambulance service was established in Alexis Creek with volunteer drivers. The service was used to transfer patients to the Cariboo Memorial Hospital in Williams Lake.

Nurse-in-charge Ms. Engelbert from Alexis Creek said, "With the ambulance service more babies were born in the ambulance than in the hospital." I can imagine women in labour in the local ambulance careening down the many switchbacks on Sheep Creek Hill to the Fraser River Bridge then up the hill and on to the hospital in Williams Lake. The trip itself would be a potent induction of labour in most pregnant women.

With the Red Cross flag out in front, the Alexis Creek Hospital has been a beacon for those seeking medical help and it has been a safe haven for all living in the frontier environment of the chilly Chilcotin plateau.

"Doc, We Got a Problem."

It was five AM Saturday, Halloween morning, when Father Michael O'Flanagan called me on the phone. "Hello, Doctor, this is Father Michael at the Indian school. Doc, we got a problem here with the boys in grade one. They've been wetting their beds most nights."

"Is this a new problem and why so early with this call? This can't be an emergency?"

I knew there was an ongoing problem every fall with the first graders wetting their beds. These little guys were taken from remote Indian reserves on the Chilcotin Plateau in central BC and sent to the Native residential schools. They were separated from their brothers and sisters and herded together in the one big dormitory. They only saw their moms and dads occasionally on long weekends. They were used to living in isolated areas where their pet dogs, kitties and horses played a big part in their lives. They were sad and at times tearful at the school. Some couldn't speak much English, which only made their loneliness worse. Many young Aboriginal women in high school made extra money by looking after the dormitories and the kids. Their supervisor was an inexperienced young nun. None of them knew what to do with the stained, stinky sheets that kept piling up in the laundry.

"These women are short of patience and out of sheets because of the bedwetting," said Father Michael.

"You know this happens every fall when the kids get lonely and homesick. This is no emergency, Father, and besides it's Halloween tonight."

"But, Doc, let me explain. This is serious. Last night the young women went to the dormitory with a spool of butcher twine."

"Butcher twine?"

"You know the thick kind that's coated with wax?"

"Yes, it's unbreakable. Joe, the butcher, uses it to wrap meat parcels when he uses that shiny brown paper."

"Yes, well, they took this tough string and tied it around six little kids' penises, below their foreskins. Now the kids are howling and their penises are swollen so bad that I can hardly see the string. They haven't peed since after supper last night."

"Father, what's going on out there? Call the ambulance and take them to the hospital now. Get some responsible nuns to go with them. Better get Sister Roberte, she has a few brains and is a nurse. Father, do not let the boys have anything to eat or drink. Do you understand?"

About thirty minutes later six little Indian boys arrived in the ambulance with Sister Roberte. They all held their genitals as the sister herded them into the emergency room.

"We've really got a mess here, Doctor. The butcher's string is strangulating their penises, but they're good kids, brave and cooperative," said Sister Roberte.

"Thanks Sister, have them take their pants and underwear off and put one in each crib. I'll see what has to be done."

One brave little boy said, "It really hurts, Doctor, and I can't pee." He rubbed his tearful dark eyes.

"Okay, son, we'll look after you all. Try not to cry and we'll get the strings cut. We'll have to put you to sleep first so we don't hurt you. The nurse will give you ice packs to put on your penises to stop the swelling. It'll be cold but be brave. We'll have to give you some needles and run some fluids into your veins. Dr. Hugh is coming to help me. He's a good guy and you all know him. He'll put a mask over your face and get you to breathe the smelly stuff and soon you'll fall asleep. When you wake up you'll be all better."

I checked each boy and noticed the knot of the string was uppermost and almost buried in the swollen foreskin. Hopefully the glands of each penis were still intact and the boys would be able to pee when the noose was removed.

After each boy was anaesthetized, I took a sharp pointed scalpel and carefully cut the fibres of the string as I squeezed the edema fluid out of the foreskin. In the recovery room, about three hours later, all the strings had been cut and ice bags covered the little boys' groins.

As the boys awakened they all wretched and there was the smell of open drop ether and vomit. Later, I asked for all of them to try and pee in the urinal so I could see the force of each stream. Then we decided to have a peeing party for the boys. The nurses, Sister Roberte and I supplied the Halloween treats to these stoic, skinny little guys. They said they'd never had a peeing party before. All the boys put on their coats and went into the vacant lot behind the hospital and stood by the edge of the road. Under an orange harvest moon each boy, in turn, peed as far as he could into the white snowbank. Chocolate bars, apples and suckers filled their parka pockets as they ran back into the hospital, each one a winner.

For the next few months my exploits were notorious at the Indian school. I was known as "the Doctor that could fix your weiner." The bedwetting didn't stop but I never had to un-noose penises again. My wife and I were invited each year, for six years, to all the school festivities. As honoured guests, we attended graduations, award nights or championship sports games held at the school.

Grace Peckinbaa from Chu-Chua

There's always one eccentric family in every frontier medical community. The Peckinbaa family filled the bill in Williams Lake. They were ruled by Grace; she was wife, mother and matriarch. The family had moved from Chu-Chua, a town located on the North Thompson River, to Soda Creek, British Columbia, in the Chilcotin region. Their stump ranch was located about twenty miles north of Williams Lake on the west side of the Fraser River. They raised sheep, poultry, cattle and kids. Roy, the father, did a little cowboying and logging when he wasn't drinking beer in the Ranch Hotel Bar in Williams Lake.

They were always known as the "Peckinbaas from Chu-Chua," even after they had moved to the Chilcotin. Grace claimed the phrase had a certain musical, poetic ring to it and was loath to give it up. She always introduced herself as "I'm Grace Peckinbaa from Chu-Chua. I raise kids, chickens and sheep."

As the new Doc in town I was assigned the families who didn't pay their bills or didn't have medical insurance. The Peckinbaa family usually arrived just before closing time on Saturday evening. They never made an appointment.

Grace was a big woman. Because of her girth and multiple pregnancies, she always wore GWG red-strap overalls, the kind with metal fasteners and brass buckles. Her "iron man pants" were tucked into cowboy boots in summer, rubber boots in winter. In the summer she didn't wear anything under her bib overalls. Grace always had a ready breast to suckle one, two or even three babes with ease in the truck.

She believed in folk cures and herbs and the opinion of Mrs. Charleyboy, the midwife for the Toosie Band on the Riske Creek Indian reserve. Mrs. Charleyboy told Grace that if she suckled her young she wouldn't get pregnant. No matter what I told Grace she always believed the midwife "what said that breast feeding stops pregnancy." Her theory that suckling babes could prevent future pregnancies failed to work nine times but she was undaunted and a loving mother nevertheless. Grace didn't believe in birth control of any kind—she said it went against her grain, whatever that meant. When I approached Roy after I had delivered their ninth child and suggested that he have a vasectomy, he replied that "no Gawd danged horse doctor is going to geld me, for only doing what come naturally."

Grace was very opinionated and always called me "Doc, Doc, you old fart, or Doc, you horse doctor," depending on her mood or the size of her medical bill.

One Saturday night, just before six PM, Grace and the kids arrived in their beat-up Chevy pickup. The towheaded brood always rode in the truck box or on the tailgate. Roy, Grace and the suckling babes all crowded into the cab. This Saturday three kids had diarrhea.

"Them kids can crap through an eye of a needle," said Grace. "They's got summer complaint."

"Really," I said.

Grace said she felt bloated and logy and her breasts were getting bigger than watermelons.

"Doc, you horse doctor, my kids is sick and I'm sicker. I'm not sure if I's bilious from them gallstones of mine with jaunders? Maybe I's got the pregnancy sickness back for the past eight months."

"You and Roy haven't been using any birth control?"

"No, Doc, I'm just nursing the two young ones. The little one is eleven months old now. My belly's been getting big, fast. It's funny, Doc, cause I'm nursing the two youngest still."

"We'll see the kids first then have a look at you. When was your last menstrual period?"

"I don't keep track no more. Probably about three years ago."

Grace was pregnant again and when I did a pelvic exam her water broke. The head was already low in the pelvis.

"Grace, you better go up to hospital—you're going to have a baby very soon. I'll phone the hospital now and tell them that you're coming. I'll be up soon."

"Are you sure, Doc?"

"Yes, I'm sure."

Grace made it to the hospital and the maternity nurse delivered yet another ten-pound towheaded Peckinbaa on the tailgate of Roy's truck. Somehow, in the confusion of the delivery, the placenta was delivered in the back of the truck and dropped onto the front step of the old shabby Williams Lake War Memorial Hospital porch. It then disappeared and the hospital administrator's golden Labrador dog didn't come home to feed for a couple of days.

"Thanks for helping me, girls," said Grace as the new baby suckled. "Does cutting and tying your tubes stop your milk from coming in, or slow it down? Expect I'll be nursing 'til the kids are all off and away in school. I think I'm going to name my son after my Doc. Sterling Peckinbaa sounds melodic, don't ya think? Maybe I'll get that there horse doctor to clip my tubes, eh?"

On yet another Saturday evening, Grace arrived sick and said "I's got the bilious colic and pain under my short ribs, goes through to my back. You told me in spring I had gallstones and needed to have 'em out. Your hospital x-rays showed hundreds of stones. But, Doc, I can't live on that low-fat diet you give me. Needs fat to keep up my strength."

"Grace, you may have to be admitted to hospital. Please stop eating fried greasy foods, now."

"Doc, forgot to tell you I've had them yellow jaunders all summer off and on. There's no way I can go to the hospital. I won't see Dr. Barney here and don't like that surgeon Doc Holy in Quesnel. Doc, you old horse doctor, I want a second opinion soon. I'm not letting them surgeons butcher me like a hog!"

"If that's the way you feel, Grace, then you'll have to go to Vancouver for the surgery."

"Geez, Doc—Vancouver? That's a long way. Doc, get me a second opinion with someone around here. I'm not going to Vancouver on your say so."

"I'll arrange someone to see you here. Now get into the examining room and put the gown on. The nurse will be in soon to help you."

I gave Grace a few moments by herself in the examining room then knocked on the door and entered.

"It hurts right here, Doc—on the right, just under my short

ribs. Don't mash me, Doc. My gut is tender."

"Grace, you're not jaundiced now but you're tender over your gall bladder. I think you have gall bladder colic from multiple gallstones. The nurse will give you a shot of Demerol. I'll try and line up a second opinion next week but be sure and get some blood work at the hospital in a day or two. Check back if you get sicker. I'll see your kids now and you next week."

On Tuesday afternoons, my afternoon off, I sometimes gave anaesthetics for the local veterinarian, Dr. John Robb. This particular Tuesday we were gelding a stallion. While infusing a pail of liquid chloral hydrate into the animal's jugular vein I had a brilliant idea.

"John, I would like you to do me a favour. Grace Peckinbaa is really sick with hundreds of gallstones but she won't see surgeon Barney Ringwood and doesn't like Dr. Holly in Quesnel. She needs surgery in Vancouver but refuses to go without a second opinion. Can I order her to your veterinarian clinic for a second opinion tomorrow? I'll send her x-rays with her."

"Sure, I'll be glad to give her a second opinion," said John with a smile on his face.

The next afternoon Roy, Grace and the kids arrived at John's veterinarian clinic on South Lakeside Drive. The Chevy pickup wheezed into the driveway and stopped. The kids piled out.

"Hi, Doc, this is my better half, Roy, and our kids. I'm Grace Peckinbaa from Chu-Chua; I raise kids, chickens and sheep. My Doc said you'd know all about my case. Oh yeah, here's the hospital x-rays in this here brown envelope."

"Let's see those x-rays, Mrs. Peckinbaa. Yes...I see you have multiple gallstones. If I were you I'd go to Vancouver and have your gall bladder out by a surgeon. That's my opinion but then I'm only a horse doctor."

DIVINITY

One Saturday night a mother, who was a member of the church of Emissaries of Divine Light, brought her sick twelve-year-old son to the emergency room of the Cariboo Memorial Hospital in Williams Lake, British Columbia. In the spring of 1961, this young mother had taken her son away from Lord Cecil (pronounced Lord Sissal) and the cult. The group had been healing her son in 100 Mile House, fifty miles (eighty kilometres) to the south. For ten days young Johnny had been receiving "atunements" but healing hands were no cure for Johnny's vomiting or the continual pain in his belly.

The mother, Mary, secretary and sometimes wife in this religious group, was frightened that her only son would die. When I saw Johnny I was in silent agreement. Mary arranged for neighbours, not associated with the Emissaries, to drive them both to the hospital. Mary knew by doing this she would be excommunicated by the Emissary Foundation. She knew Lord Cecil would be angry and she was weeping when they arrived.

"How long has Johnny been sick?" I asked. "Ten days you

said with vomiting? My God, woman, what were you thinking? He looks as dehydrated as a prune."

"I thought he was sick," Mary sobbed. "But our leader Lord Sissal, named by the group 'Uranda,' said I'd been babying him too much and that this spiritual group of male elders was going to make a man of him, if I couldn't."

The boy was incoherent, his eyes sunken, his lips parched and his abdomen distended. He was moaning. He had tenderness especially in the right lower quadrant of his abdomen.

"Hi, Johnny," I said. "You are a pretty sick boy. You're going to have some needle pricks and we are going to run some salt and sugar water into your vein with some antibiotics. We may have to take some blood from your arm as well. Don't be afraid, okay?"

"Okay, Doctor," was Johnny's feeble reply.

"Mary, I'll have to call the surgeon. Johnny has a ruptured appendix, high fever and a large appendiceal abscess. He is badly dehydrated and needs a few quarts of fluid—we'll run the fluid through his veins. To stop the infection we'll give him a couple of antibiotics through the fluid."

"I knew these people were not helping," said Mary. "My sister said Lord Sissal was appointed by God and was a member of the House of Lords in England. Lord Sissal, whose last name is Exeter, controlled the church. The railroad station for the PGE [Pacific Great Eastern] Railroad in 100 Mile House is known as the Exeter Station. The Lord and his son Michael are rich; they own half the town. I trusted him, was his secretary but he would have let my son die if we hadn't run away," she sobbed. "Oh God help us."

"As soon as your son has had four or five quarts of fluid intravenously I will ask Dr. Barney to drain the abscess. We will have to give him open drop ether to put him to sleep. He will have large rubber drains left in his abdomen to drain the pus. Later when everything settles down we can take his appendix out. He'll likely have to stay here for awhile. Prepare yourself for a long stay in town."

The huge abdominal abscess was drained under anaesthesia by the surgeon and large drains were left in his peritoneal cavity. Soon after, the young lad perked up and in a few days had charmed the other patients with his quick wit. Johnny was a sweet boy with marvelous musical talent. He was a boy soprano and knew a large selection of religious music and a few Bach cantatas; his voice could be heard throughout the wards. His lilting, pure, head tone and songs and lullabys seemed to put the babies to sleep in the nursery and women in labour at ease. His singing of "Steal Away" brought tears to the eyes of hard-bitten ranchers. He sang to the elderly Indian patients, new moms and chronic complainers.

When I had time I would pop back to the hospital at night and play checkers and, later, chess with him. Johnny soon started to eat and wander around the wards of the cramped little country hospital. After weeks his abdomen stopped draining pus and his peritoneal drains were removed.

One of the other patients at this time was Mac, a tough guy who had sustained a bullet wound to his right hip. The .30-30 had shattered the bone and he was in axis traction. His temper and vocabulary were legendary. After Mac had thrown his full, foul bedpan on the floor for the third time Johnny had a talk with him.

"If you want toilet paper, just ask me but please don't throw the stinky pan on the floor, Mac. I won't wipe your bum but I will take the pan away. If you don't like dinner please don't turn it upside down on your bed; it makes such a mess that we then have to clean up."

In a week everyone knew Johnny, his songs and his winning ways. His presence made the hospital happy. To this day, when I hear the song "Steal Away, Steal Away to Jesus" I remember Johnny, his boyish ways and the songs he sang to tame Mac and the rest of the patients in the wards.

Once Johnny was well enough to leave I brought his history of abuse by the Emissaries of Divine Light of 100 Mile House to the attention of the police and the Social Welfare Department. A few months later Sergeant Dan phoned me to say, "Lord Cecil was given a reprimand and Johnny and his mother Mary are now living in Vancouver."

Later his mother phoned me from Vancouver to say, "Johnny is doing well at school and impressing everyone with his voice and his musical talent. His rendition of 'Steal Away' remains divine."

Cut Proud

The squad car's siren stopped at the emergency room at the Cariboo Memorial Hospital in central British Columbia. The lights on the top of the squad car were casting red and blue shadows on the white snow. The light of dawn unhooked the shadows and suddenly the sun appeared.

"Geez, Doc, get a move on. Hope you got your bag, surgical set and bottled IV fluids," shouted the sergeant. "We got big trouble at the Sugar Cane Reserve."

"Keep your shirt on, Sarge, and your tunic too. You sound uptight, collar too snug? What's up?"

"Hop in, Doc, put all the stuff in the back. We got about twelve miles to go, the young constable and the chief are at the scene of the crime—waiting and scared shitless. 'The goose' in his ambulance will meet us out there. He sounded hungover when I phoned him ten minutes ago. But what else is new? Hope he doesn't get lost—they call him the goose but he can't tell north from south. Some goose."

"What's up?"

"It's a long story, Doc. Two young guys in town have been terrorizing the young Sugar Cane Indian girls. One of the guys is the hotel owner's twenty-one-year-old son and he thinks he's God's gift to women. You know him, Doc. I talked to the dad and the kid and the mayor. The dad says his son 'has been horny as hell since puberty.' The mayor says 'it's his nature.' I haven't been able to get through to the dad or the kid all this fall. I think that the Indians 'de-natured' him and another young guy when they caught 'em teepee crawling this morning at Sugar Cane."

"Sounds kinda nasty, Sarge. Can you tone down that siren—it's giving me a headache."

"Geez, Doc, I thought you were tough—just put up with it. We got real trouble in Williams Lake. If what the young constable said is right, we got a fall in the scrotums but no rise in the penises."

"You think those young braves castrated those two Lotharios?"

"Sure sounded like it to me. We may have two new eunuchs to deal with. Those Indians are great cowboys—they all know how to geld a stallion. Wouldn't think these two been 'cut proud,' though. There'll be no hormones left in their empty saddle bags."

"I agree. I'm sure those four oysters are sitting in a bucket somewhere. Hope the bleeding has stopped. Hope they didn't cut the penis—if they did it could be murder instead of just a castration or circumcision. Sarge, you better step on it."

"Geez, Doc, five minutes ago you were complaining about the noise. Now it's 'step on the gas'—make up your mind. Sure glad I got your attention. You must be thinking of pruning shears too."

I looked down at the speedometer. We were doing 120 miles (190 kilometres) an hour, dipsy-doodling around the many bends surrounding Williams Lake. I tightened my lap belt and thought

about what I would need at the scene and if I had forgotten anything. The sarge's jaw was clenched as he slowed down—careful
not to miss the turnoff to Sugar Cane. He hit the cattle guard
with a thump and my head hit the roof of the squad car.

"Sorry, Doc, we'll be there in a few minutes. I can see car
lights in the trees by Joe Geld's place, think that's where we'll
find them all. Looks like there's some onlookers, mostly young
braves and the car from the Catholic Mission. If the nurse Sister
Roberte is there things will be in good hands, so to speak. She'll
have everything under her thumb…I mean control."

We jumped out of the car. Sister Roberte and the constable
were attending the victims. I could see blood on two giant fir
trees. Bloody ropes were still wound around both trees.

"Hi, Sister, and you too, Constable. It looks like the spermatic artery may be spurting. I'll give you a hand, Sister, as soon as
I start the IVs and run a lot of fluid into both of them. I brought
three or four hemostats with me; we'll clamp and tie off the big
vessels."

"Doctor, the pulses on both of them are fast. They've lost a
lot of blood but we seem to have slowed the bleeding down now.
They were naked when we got here, tied and spread-eagled
against the trees. We cut the ropes and then covered them with
some old horse blankets. When those blankets were covered
with blood too we used my towels to control the bleeding."

"Yeah, Doc, them lariats were slippery," said the chief. "And
I couldn't get the knots loose. Sent Mac, here, to phone yous
guys from his place. Then we had to cut them new ropes—
what a waste of good lariats. Geez, Doc, that was my best
horse blanket too."

"Was there anyone around when you got here?" the sarge asked.

"There were a bunch of men with masks on running through

the trees, maybe ten. Couldn't identify any of them."

"Did you see anyone, Constable, or you, Chief?" quizzed the sarge.

"Just saw shadows running when I arrived. Couldn't identify anyone," said the policeman.

"Geezze guys, didn't see nobody," said the chief. "Only heard these two guys screaming how they'd lost their crown jewels. There was blood everywhere so I cut 'em down. That cop there and Sister laid them down and they got the horse blankets out the back of my Chevy pickup. Son-of-a-gun, they took my new blankets and covered them up. Sister had some cloths and stopped the blood from coming by stuffing them into them empty nut sacks."

"Are you sure you didn't recognize anyone, Chief?"

"Sarge, it was dark—didn't see nothin' for sure. Only seen ten or twelve shadowy-lookin' guys and anyway, Sarge, I's got a bad memory for faces."

"Later on today I want everyone to come to the station house and sign a statement."

"Geez, sarge. I can't sign nothing."

"You know more than you're saying, Chief."

"I can't read or write but I'll make my mark about these two white guys. Some guy's gelded them good. Didn't even cut 'em proud. Took all four oysters and threw the bloody things in that old leaky pail over there. Suppose you'll want to take 'em with you to make something out of it. Honest, Sarge, just tryin' to be a good Injun. Helpin' the cops and all."

"No no, Chief, we'll sort of pickle them in formaldehyde. Leave 'em in a bottle for evidence and I'll send them to the doctor pathologist in Kamloops."

"Them balls is no good now is they, Doc? Them saddle bags is empty now, I guess? Here's the goose now. Us Injuns will help you get these guys onto the stretcher and into the ambulance."

"Thanks Chief."

"See, Doc, we wouldn't hurt nobody. The Catholic Mission, the Injun Agent and the Injun Affairs knows us all as 'honest Injuns.' We don't talk much but we're honest."

The trial for these two young men went on and on. The Indian Agent supported the chief and the band. The Indian Affairs Department followed federal protocol and moved at a snail's pace. The sensational headlines in the *Williams Lake Tribune* and the *Vancouver Sun* gradually stopped. The two young men moved out of town to the Fraser Valley and teepee crawling on the reserve stopped abruptly. The case is still unsolved after all these years.

Every Halloween, a group of Indians gather together on the reserve to geld all white stallions. The horses are driven into the corral with lariats and castrated with razor-sharp knives. The chief says, "We always gelds 'em proud."

Bloody Business with a Safety Pin

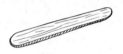

Baron Karl Friedrich Freiherr von Münchhausen (1720–1797) was a German army officer and storyteller. He embellished his adventures with tall tales, believing this would bring him fame and it did, eventually, 150 years later.

In 1951 Richard Asher coined the term Munchausen's syndrome to describe a condition in which a patient repeatedly feigns severe illness, and subjects himself to invasive medical testing in order to be hospitalized.

My first experience with Munchausen's syndrome was in Williams Lake, BC, in 1964. A young man appeared in the emergency room at midnight complaining that he had had crampy pain over his kidneys off and on for weeks and that his urine was bloody. He was asked for a urine sample and it was definitely bloody. X-rays were then taken of his abdomen and a closed safety pin was seen over his right buttock. He was given Demerol for pain management.

An intravenous pyelogram (IVP) examination in the morning revealed no kidney stones but the same safety pin was seen in different positions. When his howls of pain alarmed the nurses he was given more and more Demerol. The x-rays were sent to the regional radiologist, Dr. Pud.

Late that afternoon Dr. Pud phoned me from Quesnel and told me that there had been two previous IVPs done on this same man. Two weeks ago an IVP had been taken in Prince George and the previous week another had been obtained in Quesnel. No stones were seen but a closed safety pin was seen on all the x-rays. Pud told me that he was suspicious this was a case of Munchausen's syndrome.

The patient became very demanding and threatening and the only thing that would placate him was a shot of Demerol. I too was convinced that this was a case of Munchausen's.

I called the RCMP and the sergeant sent two huge policemen to the hospital. I met them in the nursing station outside the patient's room. They told me the patient was a drug addict and that there was a warrant out for his arrest on charges of armed robbery.

I went into the patient's room and accused him of falsifying his medical history in order to get Demerol. When I questioned him about hiding the closed safety pin he became very agressive. Just then the two policemen entered the room and took charge.

Later we pieced our evidence together and realized that he had been hiding the closed safety pin in his rectum. When asked for a urine or stool sample, he would surreptitiously remove the pin, prick his finger and place the blood in his sample. The safety pin was then returned to its hiding place in his rectum to await the next episode of urinary bleeding or bloodied stool.

The struggling patient was escorted to the paddy wagon by

the two competent policemen. He was charged with armed robbery and public mischief.

For months the nurses and I were asked repeatedly by the medical records clerk for the "condition on discharge please?" Each time we would write "in handcuffs and leg irons."

A Mickey Finn

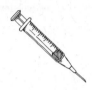

G iving an anaesthetic to a stallion can be a bit risky. If horses could read my mind it would be downright dangerous. Stallions have been known to kick and bite when confronted by a gas passer like me. It might be doubly dangerous if a horse knew what castration entailed.

Tuesday afternoons were my afternoons off duty. Sometimes, I took a busman's holiday. As a GP anaesthesiologist, I usually gave two or three anaesthetics at the Memorial Hospital in the morning. My afternoons were free to put horses, cows or dogs to sleep at the local veterinarian office. The surgeon was my friend Dr. John Robb.

For any procedure involving a horse, a horse halter and non-abrasive strong cotton ropes are essential. A serene, unhurried manner, a bucket of oats and many apples in your pocket take the place of preoperative medication. A snubbing post or hobbles should be available just in case.

One sunny August Tuesday afternoon, John picked me up at home in his Land Rover. We bumped along the gravel road to the lake pasture. We were going to Sam's paddock. Sam's stallion, his pride and joy, was going to be castrated and, while the horse was under, its umbilical hernia was to be repaired as well.

The site was chosen in the field and raked clear of firewood, cow pies and horse buns. Then a clean tarpaulin was placed centrally and John mixed up a bucket of chloride of lime and soap to wash his hands and arms. We had a "sterile field"...sort of. In a different pail I mixed up a solution of chloral hydrate: the first part of a Mickey Finn. The pail had a spout at the bottom, and attached tightly to the spout was a rubber tube, which was clamped.

Kenny, Sam's strong-looking son, went with a halter and oats to get the horse. Sam wasn't there; he preferred not to watch.

Kenny led the horse to the centre of the tarp. In a special way, John tied the soft cotton ropes to the horse's neck and legs. The plan was to gently ease the stallion onto the canvas tarp as the horse slowly lost consciousness from the anaesthetic.

I readied my equipment. My laryngoscope, which was fashioned in Joe's machine shop, had a notch for my right foot. The curved blade resembled the curve of a human Macintosh laryngoscope. A large piece of one-inch garden hose was to be used as an endotracheal tube, if necessary. I moved the pail of chloral hydrate solution close to the animal's neck.

Whap! I hit the animal's jugular vein with a number 12 needle. Blood spurted; I was in the vein. The rubber tubing was attached to the needle and I began titrating chloral hydrate into the vein. Slowly the horse became wobbly and with the ropes we gently eased the stallion down on his side. Then I extended the horse's neck, grabbed the tongue with a clamp and pulled it forward. The respirations were even and the airway partially secured; the surgeon could begin.

The spermatic cord and vessels were clamped in a flash. The two oysters soon lay on the ground, oozing in the sun.

John then started on the "vest over pants" umbilical hernia repair. It was hard to tell the vest from the pants but eventually the silk sutures pulled everything together.

There seemed to be an extra bit of "pants" left over but the hernia had been repaired. Slowly the horse woke up and re-gained its feet. A whack on the butt and he fled the recovery space in a gallop. Ah! Sweet success.

Years later I could always tell that same gelding. If he saw me he would whinny, his eyes would flash and he'd run to the end of the field. When I looked at his belly button I could see a bit of "pants," like a miniature second penis extending from a flat belly.

At home that night I completed the Mickey Finn by enjoying a few drams of Irish whisky.

* A Mickey Finn is a strong alcoholic drink, which in this case refers to a combination of whisky and chloral hydrate.

Tick Paralysis

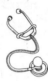

It was during the dog days of summer, 1963, in the Cariboo region of British Columbia that I saw my first case of tick paralysis. The second case was seen a few weeks later.

The emergency room of the dilapidated rural hospital in Williams Lake was abuzz after the Williams Lake Stampede, an annual July 1 event. The dust was slowly settling down after a week of drinking, steer decorating, saddle bronc busting, calf roping, quarter horse races and accidents. The First Nations people loaded their kids and summer supplies in their cayuse-pulled covered wagons and with their quarter horses trailing, they headed home across the Fraser River for the Chilcotin.

My first tick paralysis patient arrived July 3. Judy was a pretty blue-eyed, six-year-old girl with thick golden braids. Her folks ran a neat and tidy motel in town but also had a small hobby ranch just west of town on the Dog Creek Road. The two kids had spent the previous five days at the ranch playing with the dogs and riding their ponies. Her mother explained, "My daughter Judy had wanted to come into town early in the morning. She had not been feeling well and had fallen down a few times. Joey, her younger brother, was still at the ranch with Dad, riding their pony, Daisy."

Usually, Judy was an alert, strong, happy young girl on the go. When I first saw her she seemed unsteady on her feet and held onto her mom for support; she complained of a funny feeling in her legs and a headache. Her mother assured me that Judy had been given Salk vaccine (an inoculation to prevent polio) at the beginning of grade one, ten months ago, and no one was sick at home. I had to find another cause of the weakness in Judy's legs now that polio had been ruled out.

My examination revealed marked weakness of her lower extremities and absent knee and ankle reflexes but little else. Her complete blood count and her spinal fluid revealed no abnormalities. Then, on a hunch, I asked the mother to undo Judy's braids and I re-examined her, starting at the top of her head.

At the back of her neck under the knot of her braid I found a large engorged female tick, a Rocky Mountain wood tick, *Dermacentor andersoni*. Her mother was flabbergasted but relieved when I explained that once I removed the tick Judy would make a full recovery from tick paralysis.

We decided to keep Judy in the hospital overnight and in the morning this sweet little girl was back to her normal self. The next morning she said she wanted to go back to the ranch to see her kitty, Tigger, and ride their pony, Daisy.

Tick paralysis is not the result of an infective agent but is due to the secretions of a neurotoxin by the blood-feeding, egg-filled, mother wood tick. In the Cariboo, there are few human cases but many cattle and sheep die of tick paralysis. The disease is well known to veterinarians.

The second case of tick paralysis was a First Nation twelve-year-old boy from the Chilcotin region. He was brought to the hospital by nurse Sister Roberte of the Alexis Creek Catholic Mission, from the Redstone Reserve. This little guy had paralysis of his lower legs and had difficulty breathing. Sister Roberte didn't think he'd had any of his immunizations and according to his grandmother, "Joey had been sick for over a week." The parents had been away salmon fishing at Farwell Canyon on the Chilcotin River since the Williams Lake Stampede, July 1.

Upon examination I confirmed that this skinny little guy had complete paralysis of his legs and had difficulty breathing. I located an engorged tick in Joey's ear. The tick had completely filled his ear canal and I had to remove the tick in small pieces. I then intubated Joey, placed an endotracheal tube in his trachea and started resuscitation with an Ambu inflatable bag. With my partner, Hugh Atwood, we bagged him for eighteen hours. The Cariboo War Memorial Hospital did not have a mechanical ventilator at this time.

Unfortunately the neurotoxin secreted by the female tick's salivary glands was in complete control of Joey by the time I removed the arachnid and despite our efforts he slowly became unresponsive. Joey died the next morning. This was a sad, rare human death from tick paralysis.

WILLOUGHBY

Many Indian kids on Chilcotin reservations are named after Charlie Willoughby, a surgeon and one-time partner of mine from Kamloops, BC. Charlie was also a politician and was elected to Parliament in Ottawa in the 1950s. His campaign trail included some isolated Native communities. On March 31, 1960, Canadian First Nations people were allowed to vote for the first time. Many of the Native men and women of the Chilcotin were thrilled at being able to cast their ballot for the first time and associated Charlie with their newly granted rights even though his campaign had ended by the time they were given the vote.

For years many Chilcotin Natives named their boys after Charlie—Willoughby Quilt had a good Anglo-Saxon sound to it and a royal ring. These boys were full-blooded Canadians as good as anybody. No more would they be called that "damned Mac Quilt."

My first meeting with Willoughby Quilt was in the maternity section in the dilapidated War Memorial Hospital's case room in Williams Lake, BC. His mother spoke mostly Chilcotin and came from Nemiah Valley. Willoughby came out of his mother's womb screaming. When I put the baby to the mother's breast, she said "Willoughby."

Willoughby lived in an isolated area, a First Nations village of about thirty log houses many miles south of Alexis Creek. In Willoughby's house there was no running water or electricity. The road in was made of mud and a corduroy of logs laid cross-ways through the swamps. This trail, at its onset, was labelled by a primitive sign that read: "This Road Is Impassable, Not Even Jackassable." This path was named the Jackass Way and it was bumpy the entire length. The Nemiah Valley in the Coast Mountains gives pasture to a large band of wild mustangs and people, both tough as rawhide.

The second time I met Willoughby was during the Williams Lake Stampede when as a nine-month-old infant he became badly dehydrated from severe diarrhea. After months in the old hospital he was taken back home by Sister Roberte from the Alexis Creek Catholic Mission. The father seemed to be too busy either hunting moose or telling hunting stories in the Alexis Creek beer parlour to bother to pick up his son and his mother was pregnant with another child. Sister Roberte returned this handsome little boy to his grandmother's tender loving care.

The last time I saw Willoughby was during a February cold snap. The public health nurse told me that she had received word that Mrs. Quilt's water had broken and she needed to come to the hospital in Williams Lake. She was just setting out for the arduous journey from Alexis Creek to Nemiah to bring her in. I told her that we'd be looking for her and to be careful driving along "Jackass Way."

About seven hours later I got a phone call from the midwife at the Alexis Creek Hospital. She said that "Mrs. Quilt was there and not in labour. The public health nurse had to go back to

Nemiah because in their haste to leave they had left Willoughby wrapped up in blankets at the foot of Quilts' bed in a Chilcotin cradle. There had been a pretty good fire going in the woodstove of the cabin when they left but it would be another three to four hours before they could rescue him."

"Did you try to phone the chief or one of the councillors?" I asked.

"Doctor, there are no telephones, just one old radio-phone in Nemiah. I'll keep you posted every few hours."

After a number of hours the nurse phoned me and related the story: While she went to fetch Willoughby, the midwife had delivered Mrs. Quilt's baby in the Alexis Creek Outpost Hospital. The mother would be coming in by ambulance in a day or two with the new baby; both were doing well. When the nurse got to the Quilts' log home it was bitterly cold and the wood fire had gone out. On searching at the foot of the bed she found Willoughby wrapped in sleeping bags and sound asleep, warm as toast. She changed his dirty diaper, gave him a bottle of milk, some banana and pablum. She then wrapped him up again in the down sleeping bag and took him with her to Alexis Creek Hospital. "We'll be back in 'The Lake' in a couple of days," she said, "you can check Willoughby over then."

Near-Death Experience

The phone rang at ten o'clock Friday morning, July 16, 2005. A woman's voice said, "Is that Doctor Haynes, who used to practise in Williams Lake, BC? This is Trish. We owned a hotel in Williams Lake, in 1964. Do you remember me and my husband, Roger, and our kids?"

The synapses in my memory made the connection rapidly. I had been her GP for fifteen years. Her husband, Roger, and son, Andy, and I played racquetball occasionally. I hadn't seen her or her family for twenty-five years.

"How could I forget you, Trish? I still have nightmares forty-two years later about you. If I remember correctly you had an ectopic pregnancy and went into shock. Is that right? And your son Andy dislocated his kneecap on the squash court?"

"What a memory, Sterling, after all these years. Yes, you fixed Andy's patella right on the court. Andy is almost fifty now and is an airline pilot. You remember the other two girls...you delivered K, the last one."

"You must be proud of your kids. Congratulations on all those grandchildren."

"I've just read your book *Bloody Practice*, Sterling. It made me want to contact you and relate the near-death experience I had during my tubal pregnancy. I have only related this experience to my family but I feel that I need to tell you as a sort of therapeutic exercise. Get it off my chest so to speak."

"Please go ahead," I told her.

"Years ago you told me that if I ever had severe abdominal pain that spread to my shoulder tip it meant something had ruptured in my abdomen. A few months ago I developed just such a pain so I went to my GP but in a few hours the pain disappeared. The ultrasound scan showed a large ovarian cyst, which after surgery was found to be a benign tumor of my right ovary. It was a big one but it had leaked a little fluid and caused the shoulder pain. My doctor said it wasn't cancer. I'm okay now but it reminded me of the near-death dreams that followed my tubal pregnancy."

"That experience influenced my dreams as well for a long time. I still remember giving you a spinal anaesthetic, which after a few minutes sent you into shock. Anaesthesia administration can be filled with hours of boredom interspersed with moments of terror. This was the case with you. I was terrified."

"This is what I remember of that experience. Dr. Donald MacLean admitted me to the hospital when I went to him because of severe abdominal pain that spread to my shoulder tip. He told me that I had an ectopic pregnancy that had ruptured and bled into my abdomen and that I would need surgery right away. Shortly after you anaesthetized me I felt myself in a long black tunnel. I resisted going there but it seemed to engulf me, overwhelm me. I woke up to hear you saying, 'She's got a belly full of blood—find the Gawd-damned blood filter so we can scoop the blood out of her belly and run it through the filter back into her. If you can't find it you better get some blood donors down here fast, she's A-positive.' I remember that you started another IV in my other arm to run more fluid into me and that the tilted operating table made me feel like I was almost standing on my head. I can remember the sound of oxygen running through my mask and your voice over the noise saying 'Talk to me, Trish. Talk to me.'"

"You can remember all those details, Trish, even now?"

"Yes I can. Han, the surgeon, said he was sweating and asked the nurses for a wipe of his brow. Then he said, 'I've got hold of her tube with my fingers...she'll be okay now.' This is probably when you said, 'Everything's under control.' The long tunnel receded in my mind and made a right turn down a black sooty stovepipe. I wanted to waken and see Roger and the kids. The darkness was shifting to a kind of grey. I could see you pumping the blood into me and everything seemed lighter second by second."

"That was a long, cold winter night, Trish. Who could forget it? Han died last year at the age of eighty; what a great guy he was. Donald is a retired psychiatric professor living in Oxford, Mississippi, now."

"I'm so sorry about Han, Sterling. I'm glad you remember that night too. Thank you for letting me recall this experience with you. This has haunted me since it happened; it's been stored in the back of my brain, coming out occasionally during death's revisiting hours."

THOMPSON
-
OKANAGAN

Hockey Night in Kamloops

About thirty-five years ago we were sitting in the change room of the old North Kamloops hockey arena in our long underwear and equipment. I was sweating and hurting. I had just collided with a young surgeon, my partner, Mike Budzinski—or was it Bud Mikinski? I was concussed and incoherent, I think.

We were playing on opposing teams in a professional league of doctors, lawyers, optometrists and dentists. There was a lot of skill amongst the players, just not for playing hockey, except for Dr. Mike—in his youth, Mike had played for the Regina Pats in the Western Junior A Hockey League.

During the game we collided near the net in my end and I crashed into a solid steel net post. Our team lost 8–0. Mike scored all the goals.

My shoulder was so sore I could hardly get my cup off and I couldn't shrug off my long combination Stanfield underwear; the wool was stuck to my hide. The room was cold, as was the water in the showers. The benches were splintery where hockey players over the years had aimlessly kicked holes with their skates. To top off the night, I ran a slender, long, fir splinter into my backside—I still bear the scar where my wife picked the sliver out with a needle and a pair of tweezers.

We were professionals, but it was not an elite hockey league. That night I thought I might retire from a life of hockey after thirty-five years as a player and team doctor. Another of my partners, Dr. Bob, thought we could make a team statement by volunteering to become doctors for the junior A team, the Kamloops Blazers.

So, for the next thirteen years Bob or I attended all the hockey games and playoffs at the Memorial Arena on Victoria Street. It was a memorable time, but we never won the Memorial Cup. We were the official team docs and sat in seats behind the players' benches. We were given two tickets to every game in payment for our services. I attended more than five hundred games before I officially resigned.

One of the first things I had to learn was the hockey lingo. The main two adjectives used to describe every conceivable hockey event are the F word and the S word. They can be used interchangeably or together as an adjective or more likely as a present participle with certain practised hockey sayings.

When the two of us were asked to comment on a game, certain phrases had to be committed to memory: "We gotta play our game; A few lucky breaks; Cud'uh gone either way; Did you see that hit?; That was a soft goal." The F word and the S word could be used before each noun except when the wives were present or when giving a commentary to the local radio stations.

One of the first problems we came across involved Joe, the Zamboni icemaker, and the young chief referee, a man with the last name of Fraser who went on to become a prominent referee in the National Hockey League. The City of Kamloops had neglected to service the Zamboni over the summer. During one of the games in October many of the players began complaining to their coaches of feeling sick or "woozy-like." The coach's answer was, "You bunch of s***heads—we need to send the lot of you back to your families in Saskatchewan and Alberta. The remainder we can ship back to Vanderhoof and Prince George to your mothers."

Then Referee Fraser collapsed in the dressing room after the second period of a league game. The administration branch of the team felt that maybe something was fishy. Especially when, during that same game, Joe kept cutting circles with his Zamboni through a haze of smoke and fumes. He finally fell off his seat on the machine onto the wet ice.

The medical staff called the ambulance for Joe and Fraser. The two of them were shipped off to the hospital for testing and oxygen inhalation treatment. The Zamboni was pushed off the ice and the double doors of both ends of the arena were opened to the frigid temperatures. The players immediately felt better in the fresh air and the play started in the third period without Joe and Fraser. Fraser stayed in the emergency room of the Royal Inland Hospital 'til midnight—he had a most severe case of carbon monoxide poisoning. It turned out that the team owners had decided in September that repairs to the Zamboni exhaust system were too expensive for the budget and should be paid for by the city. The rapacious executive officer said, "Then what the hell, if the city is not going to fix the f***ing machine, then neither will the owners."

It was at this time that I realized major decisions about the team were left to local ex-hockey players and businessmen on the "old boy" executive. Money was the bottom line, even though the Kamloops team was a farm team and had an agreement with the wealthy New York Islanders of the NHL. To me, these economic decisions were made by people who "had their bell rung too many times, or had blocked too many slapshots with their teeth."

Through the many years, Dr. Bob, Dr. Gord and I looked after fractures, dislocated joints and thousands of lacerations and hematomas. All the suturing was done at the end of the game in the two dressing rooms. We brought our own sterile surgical trays from our offices.

There was no payment and little thanks from the Blazers' executive. Most of the young hockey players were polite and appreciative, and it was a pleasure to work with them and applaud their skills on the ice. For the most part, I got along with the coaches until an incident at the end of the 1979 season, when a young player from the Regina Pats complained to me after the game.

"Doc, I don't feel good...sweating all the time, no energy and I'm getting all these knots in my neck. I had a sore throat for a while but that got better. I told the coach but he told me to smarten up, the playoffs are just around the corner. 'Do you want to go back to Lucky Lake, Saskatchewan?' I'm only sixteen and I'm the leading scorer on the team and he's making fun of me and cursing me."

"Yes, I know you are a great player. You take off your equipment, have a shower and then I'll examine you in the medical room here. How tall are you?"

"I'm six foot three inches. Been going to school and working on the farm all my life. My dad says I'm worth two hired men and that I'm still growing."

I examined the young giant and found he had infectious mononucleosis and a very large spleen associated with mild hepatitis. Lab tests confirmed the diagnosis.

I held a meeting with the team executive and the coaches the next evening. Then I told them, "This young man cannot play for at least six weeks, maybe longer. If his enlarged spleen ruptured from a hard check or even a butt end from a stick, he could die without emergency surgery."

"What if you're f***ing wrong, Doc?" asked the coach.

Two days later I found out that the coaches and the executive had insisted this young man play, "no matter what." They had disregarded my advice.

The young player phoned me from Calgary to tell me that the coach made him play. He told me, "I felt bad, real bad but the coach played me the whole game."

I contacted the league president and then phoned his mother and father in Lucky Lake. I told his mother her son's coaches and management were jeopardizing his life and health. His mom thanked me and told me her son would recuperate at home for six weeks. There would be lots of home cooking for this well-loved gentle giant.

This same player became an all-star centre-ice man for the St. Louis Blues hockey team. He played for twenty-one years in the NHL and became a hall-of-famer.

That same year, the Kamloops Blazers made the playoffs. When I went to pick up my tickets for the first game, I found they had been sold and the team president said they'd "do without a doctor during the playoffs or maybe find somebody else to fill in. The new doctor could stand in the players' bench."

I had been fired for calling the player's parents, kicked out of my sacred hockey pew. It was time to become a father to my four loving daughters and a full-time husband and doctor.

My life in hockey ended, but I occasionally meet with my old buddies over a beer. During these discussions I am always reminded of the dressing room quip by great writer and old-time hockey player for the University of Waterloo Worriers, Ted Mc-Gee: "The older I get the better I was."

The Murphy Bed

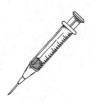

Terence Flanagan was a lovable reprobate who resided in old hotels and cheap motels. In 1970, he was living in a motel on Victoria Street in downtown Kamloops, BC. He was a semi-retired, aging jockey who still managed to ride a few mounts in the central British Columbia race circuit, which included the Williams Lake Stampede, Kamloops' Sagebrush Downs and Vernon's Kin Park. Terry had been born in the slums of Dublin, Ireland, and had been poorly fed as a child. Rickets had caused the bony rachitic rosary of his chest and his bow legs were due to lack of vitamin D. As a child, his small stature and bandy legs made him an ideal exercise boy.

One hot summer morning, Terry was brought into the emergency room by two medics. The motel room where Terry had been lodging had developed a strong smell. The stink had upset the guests of the motel and they complained to the manager. Terry had placed a "Do Not Disturb" sign on the handle of his door after he had checked in, drunk, twelve hours before. The odour emanating from the room was so intense that the night clerk disregarded the sign and used his master key to open the door. The room was in disarray and the foul smell made the clerk flinch. Glancing around he saw Terry hanging from the top of the Murphy bed moaning, his head compressed between the bed spring and the wall frame. The clerk called 911 and then the cops.

Terry's first words to me in the emergency room were: "I had an accident with me Murphy bed."

"An accident with a Murphy bed? You are full of the blarney, Terence Flanagan."

"It's like this, Doc. I'd tied one on good a couple of days ago after I rode a big winner. I was up on Irish Mist—a long shot at 20–1. The race was a mile and a sixteenth for four-year-old geldings who hadn't won in six months. I knew me horse had one bad leg so I put bute in his oats that morning."

"Bute?"

"You know butazolidin? It helps with me mounts' joint pains. It also makes me horses run faster."

"Then what happened?"

"That Irishman gelding took off. And we won by four lengths. I made four hundred bucks. Me friends and I went to Kelly O'Bryan's Bar and Grill and we celebrated with Irish whisky. Then me friends sent me back to the motel in a cab."

"Go on."

"Well, Doc, it starts to get complicated. I started vomiting and fell on top of this Murphy bed. I hadn't taken my cowboy boots off and when trying to get them off the heel of my boot caught on the spring-loaded catch to the bed. Somehow me head got squeezed between the sagging spring and the steel bar of me bed at the same time. I got a quick spring-loaded ride into the wall. Me bed's counterweights held me fast. The pointed toes of me boots gave me a bit o' support on the floor. Like a puppet, hanging there, I was."

"Oh my God, Terry."

"It was a long night after that. The Murphy bed wedged me head tighter between the spring and the frame. Being so light I couldn't overpower the wall spring that held me upright, like hanging I was, by me skull. Luckily me toes just touched the ground."

"Didn't you try and get out or call for help?"

"I couldn't reach the catch to let the bed down and there was a big party in the next unit so I knew they wouldn't hear me hollering. My neck was really twisted and all. I couldn't help myself, Doc, the next thing I knew all the beer and whisky came back up and what was left over came out from me bladder. I was a stinking mess."

"I can imagine. How long were you held up like this?"

"Must have been over ten hours. Was I glad to see those medics. They had to use 'the jaws of life' to cut me out from the bedspring."

Terry had a huge pressure defect along the side of his ear and his head from the pressure of the frame and the spring. Already the area was infected. I got some x-rays of his skull and neck to see if there was a fracture. Then I froze the area and cut out some of the infected scalp and tried to refashion part of the top of his ear.

"Am I going to live, Doc?"

"You may end up with a bit of a cauliflower ear but your x-rays look okay. You understand that with pressure plus infection in the cartilage your ear will be permanently deformed. We'll clean you up and get some decent clothes for you before we let you go in a day or two."

"Okay Doc, let's get started. Well, I learned a good lesson. Whisky and Murphy beds just don't mix."

Terry was kept in hospital for a couple of days of IV antibiotics and ice packs to reduce the swelling. He was a model patient in the hospital but was anxious to get to the track and horse barn to see all his four-legged and two-legged friends. When he was discharged his right ear was a swollen, bruised, deformed piece of skin and cartilage. At his recheck, twelve days later, Terry told me he'd turned over a new leaf and from now on he'd drink only Kokanee beer. No more Bushmill's Irish Whisky.

Months later at the Sagebrush Downs I spotted Terry in his racing silks. I knew it was Terry because his racing helmet was lopsided; it wouldn't fit over his cauliflower right ear. He was walking his horse and on the large betting board, Irish Mist was a 40–1 long shot.

I went to the crowded paddock to see Terry saddle up. I gave him a wave as he rode by. He saw me and gave me a wink and a thumbs-up. The horse was a beauty, walking easily. Had the gelding had a morning breakfast of "bute" and oats, I wondered?

"The Mist" left the starting gate in the lead, ran the one-mile and one-eighth and set a track record. I have to admit, I did place a small wager on the gelding. After all, who can resist the luck of the Irish?

TONY

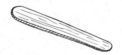

Many years ago MDs had a problem collecting their fees in money. Some debts were paid for with sacks of potatoes and turnips, eggs in water glass, pickled hog feet, chickens, moose steaks and pig carcasses. Once, in payment for delivering a healthy baby, a big game guide and hunter deposited a four-point buck, neatly dressed, in my medical waiting room.

When I had a chance to become the CNR doctor I jumped at the opportunity. Not only would I be paid by CNR cheques but the CNR would also send me many of their Workers' Compensation cases, which paid well and on time. Besides a guaranteed paycheque, I received a free railway pass and my family paid half-fare for their trips. No longer would I have to appear in small claims court on Saturday morning, fighting to collect even a portion of my outstanding fees.

One of the first people I met once I started working for the CNR was a bright, young translator. His name was Tony and he was eleven years old. Tony was gifted; he spoke excellent English and superb Italian.

Though not formally trained at this time, Tony proved to be an excellent psychologist. He had an intimate knowledge of the comings and goings of everyone in his Italian community and first-hand knowledge of all the CNR jobs and all workers on the B and B and the extra-gangs. These short, swarthy Italian men kept the track in order, restoring the main line after destruction from train wrecks, mountain rock slides and avalanches. In the middle of winter there were many accidents and I was often called to the emergency room. I quickly got to know the men and gradually their families; I delivered babies and looked after the kids. I was known as Mister Doctor.

The school kids were all fluent in English but many of the Italian women learned very little English and remained isolated in their Italian community. Tony was a gem. He was my personal translator after four o'clock every day when school was out. Pregnant bodies, infidelity or drunkenness never embarrassed him. Tony always knew when to leave my office after translating and was never embarrassed by stories of a sexual nature, except once.

One day, a young, beautiful, married Italian woman, who spoke only Italian, requested to be fitted for a diaphragm. After the birth of her third child she had lost faith in the rhythm method of birth control recommended by the Catholic bishop in our diocese. I had asked Tony to help translate the appointment before I realized the patient wished to have the diaphragm fitted that very visit.

In my office I brought out my large plastic model of the female pelvic regions and my assortment of different sizes of diaphragm fitting rings. I tried to explain to my patient about the use of the diaphragm and spermicidal jelly but she didn't seem to understand. I was going to have to rely on Tony, the teenager, to discuss the use and application of this method of birth control.

With characteristic steadiness, he translated my explanation of the fitting of the rubber ring while I demonstrated on the manikin. I asked Tony to explain that the diaphragm would only be an effective method of birth control if it were correctly placed and the way to determine this was to feel for the cervix; it would feel like touching the tip of one's nose. At this point, Tony became ashen and excused himself from my office.

My nurse then took the patient into the examining room for the actual fitting of the ring and the diaphragm. I am certain that the patient never did understand that her cervix, when touched, felt like the tip of her nose.

For seven years Tony was the official translator for the doctors in the medical clinic in Kamloops, BC. It was only when he'd grown into a man and graduated from the University of British Columbia as a teacher and a councillor that we realized what a valuable asset he had been to all twenty-seven doctors in our medical practice as well as to the Italian community. In retrospect, I realized what a great talent Tony had and wasn't surprised to learn that he later became a psychologist in the local school system.

LEO

I have come to know that some men are inherently evil. Leo was a young man with no redeeming features. He was a heroin addict and a trafficker in cocaine, LSD and barbiturates. When I met him he was on parole from Ontario's notorious Kingston Penitentiary. His major crime was armed robbery and assault with a claw hammer. He had scalped and clawed an elderly Chinese grocery store owner during the robbery.

After Leo served his ten years he stayed in Kingston getting into trouble as a drug trafficker and for his involvement in petty crime. The story goes that finally the police and city fathers gave this ex-con a one-way bus ticket to Kamloops, BC. In the 1970s this type of action by cops and city aldermen was a common way of ridding a city of unwanted, unsavoury hoods from the downtown core.

As physicians, my colleague Bernie and I looked after the AA Society members in Kamloops, BC. Both of us tried on many occasions to enlist the help of our medical colleagues but many didn't want to be called to the police station at three AM. Some of the older Docs just gave the addicts what they wanted when they appeared in their offices during office hours—get the addict out the door with their prescription for morphine, Seconal, valium or whatever, seemed to be their attitude. Street drug users were well aware of the doctors who were available for prescriptions. Within the AA Society, Bernie and I knew the addicts as well as the docs who gave out prescriptions at their demand.

An eighty-three-year-old practising physician referred Leo to me. This bozo was sent to me for counselling and possible inclusion in the methadone drug replacement program. He appeared at noon at the back door of the clinic demanding that I see him. Leo wanted a repeat of one hundred Dilaudid pills and two hundred Seconal, "them red babies" as Leo called them. I tried to enlist him in the methadone treatment plan but he refused my plan just as I refused his request. After a heated argument he left the clinic without the prescription. He appeared many times over the next few weeks, always demanding Dilaudid and Seconal and I always refused.

Leo finally left the medical clinic with a curse. He promised me that if he couldn't get his drugs legally he would "get me" and my family. This was the beginning of a long vendetta that lasted two years. Somehow, Leo obtained the city and clinic on-duty call list and knew the nights when I would be busy.

Our doctor-patient relationship ended when Leo started phoning my wife, Jesse, when I was on-call and not available at home. Over the phone he threatened my wife, saying that he would kidnap one or two of our youngest daughters from school, take them to the Thompson River and drown them. We immediately notified the RCMP and the teachers at Beattie Elementary School. Our children were placed on a strict curfew right away. If the kids were away from home we always knew where they were.

When I phoned the RCMP the sergeant in charge said their

hands were tied, it was Leo's word against mine. Two young constables interviewed Leo but he denied everything. The police by this time knew he was an addict and a pusher and knew of his violent past. He was kept on partial police surveillance but his phone threats of violence against our daughters still continued to my wife when I was on-call, away from home.

Then two plainclothes policemen devised a method of entrapment. They bugged one of my examining rooms and my main office and then positioned themselves in the examining room. Leo usually hung around the clinic about noon so when everything was in place to record our conversation I asked Leo to come into my office to discuss his drug problem. Leo was eager to oblige as he thought he might get more Dilaudid from me. The interview I had with Leo in my private office was a great success. Leo admitted that he was constantly threatening to murder our children but stated that this would stop if I would give him a continuous source of prescription drugs. After hearing Leo's confession the two young policemen in the next room burst into my office and arrested him. Within three hours Leo was out on a ten thousand dollar bail and remanded.

The trial was scheduled to be held in Vernon in two months' time but while we waited for the court date Leo still kept uttering threats to my wife and me. This time he said he was going to murder all four of our daughters.

This terrorizing continued at a stepped-up pace all summer and fall even when he was remanded and placed under partial police surveillance. Jessie and I felt helpless; all we could do was watch our four daughters even more carefully. We drove them everywhere and notified our close friends and neighbours to be on the alert for suspicious people on our street. Our daughters were angry at all the restrictions we placed on them. We were all sleepless and bad tempered and had many emotional outbursts at the dinner table. Things were even worse when I was on-call and away from home at night. My wife and I became more watchful and more angry; by now our surveillance was all consuming and interfering with our family's life.

It was a cold, slushy, November day when Jessie and I arrived at the county courthouse in Vernon. We were immediately ushered in to the police office in the courthouse. The police sergeant told us that Leo had enlisted a highly successful Vancouver criminal lawyer to defend him. I thought that the prosecutor for the crown might call me but by ten AM he still had not arrived at the courthouse to give us instructions. When the prosecuting lawyer finally did arrive it was obvious the man had not prepared anything. He was late and knew little about the case.

Leo's lawyer from Vancouver appeared well groomed in a grey silk suit. He spoke very well and obviously knew the ins and outs of the case. He appeared to know Leo well, having defended him in the past. The case was over within an hour. The two young constables had charged Leo under the wrong act of the criminal code.

By eleven AM the case was thrown out, case dismissed. Leo was free to go. As we filed out, I was following Leo and he turned to me and said, "F.O., Doc."

His threats against our daughters continued until Christmas Eve. After seeing my final patient that evening I was leaving the clinic when I spied a short burly man waiting by the back door. It was Leo and as usual, he demanded two hundred Dilaudid tablets. I suggested we talk outside the clinic in the alley, adding, "I will have my prescription pad with me."

I was in a rage and once we were in the darkened alley I picked Leo up and threw him into the dumpster. He came out spluttering, covered with garbage and slime. I threw him in again and this time threatened to break both kneecaps with a tire wrench. He stayed in the dumpster and remained silent. I walked away to my vehicle in the parking lot. As I drove off my car headlights picked up the shadow of a stocky man running down the alley.

I never saw or heard from Leo again. Perhaps the Kamloops city fathers and the RCMP provided him with a free one-way bus ticket back to Kingston.

SPOONEY

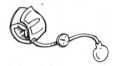

The word "spoon" is derived from the old English word *spon* meaning chip of wood or piece of carved horn used as an eating utensil. The development and uses of the spoon have been amazing.

In the late eighteenth century, to be a spoon or spooney was slang for simpleton. Thanks to the luck of the on-call doctor, I came to understand that lost meaning both viscerally and physically. In August 1972, my medical duties included servicing the provincial jail in Kamloops, British Columbia, the very month that a number of inmates decided to protest the use of "the hole" as a method of punishing prisoners who had attacked guards.

The provincial jail occupied an old World War II military camp and armory on the edge of Kamloops, on a hill overlooking the North Thompson River. This wind-swept, grey jail converted from old army barracks was ringed by a chain-link fence wound with razor wire. It was a bleak, desolate place set among sagebrush, rabbit bush and prickly pear cactus. "The hole" was a concrete cell without windows, twelve feet by twelve feet, buried in the ground, in a cellblock in the centre of the jail. The cell was accessible by a ladder, which extended fourteen feet below, to the cold, damp, concrete floor. A 20-watt bulb lit the hole. The guards lowered bread, water and porridge to the prisoner below. The slop pail was usually emptied daily through a steel grate in the ceiling. The sentence for attacking a guard could be up to one week in solitary confinement.

The prisoners frequently complained about the hole and the food. In the jail there were three times as many spoons as forks or knives. The spoons were given to the difficult prisoners to use at mealtimes but there was no spoon count at the end of meals as the instrument was thought to be innocuous. The inmates, in August 1972, proved the warden's reasoning wrong.

Many of the young men kept their spoons and took them to the metal workshop where prisoners stamped out new licence plates. Hacksaws were easily available here as were files, which could be used to smooth the edge of the handle once it had been cut off. The handle of the spoon could then be easily swallowed or pushed up a rectum.

It was my week on-call to see after-hour medical complaints of prisoners. There were the usual complaints of indigestion, constipation and abdominal pain. Prisoners are the greatest thesbians in the world—they can all give command performances.

One evening I was besieged by several plaintive complaints in the jail's medical room, a late night prisoner's sick parade. "Doc, you gotta do something. I swallowed a spoon handle. My ass is on fire, on fire, Doc. What are you going to do about it, Doc?"

Sometimes the modified spoon handle got obstructed in the prisoner's stomach. When that happened the surgeon would remove the spoon from the patient's stomach with a flexible gastroscope in the hospital. Other times the sawed-off spoon would be lodged in the rectum and with the aid of a sigmoido-scope and using large Kelly or ring forceps, I would pluck the spoon out of the rectum in the emergency room. Occasionally I had to use well-lubricated, small "sugar tong" obstetrical forceps to remove the spoon handle when it was stuck crossways within the rectum.

Orderlies at the jail sometimes gave numerous laxatives and enemas in order to hasten the passage of spoon handles. This didn't seem to deter the men in their complaint for change of food and punishment "in the hole." In fact, none of these painful consequences seemed to deter the men in their manner of pro-test. The supply of spoon handles seemed limitless.

One evening, a week after my first introduction to the pro-testing prisoners, a modified spoon perforated the colon of a young man. I called the surgeon and he performed a colostomy that night. The prisoner had a very stormy postoperative course with fever and pain. The administration of IV fluids and naso-gastric suction via a large tube in the stomach lasted for a week. After two weeks in the Royal Inland Hospital the man was sent back to the four-bed infirmary at the Kamloops jail. There I con-tinued to look after his long-term needs and his colostomy care and colostomy bags. I returned the spoon handle, labelled "Prop-erty of the BC Government," to the warden.

Word soon got around the jail's exercise yard that swallowing modified spoons could be detrimental to your health. If it didn't kill you it could mean that you'd be forced to shit in a bag for months, if not life. After the colostomy catastrophe, the illegal stealing and swallowing of government spoons ceased.

All participants in this lark had silver-coloured spoon handles drawn on the front of their medical charts so that fu-ture MDs who served on the jail's medical roster would be fore-warned. These charts also recorded the prisoner's history, his on-command theatrical performances and his spooney she-nanigans.

It wasn't 'til the new jail was built, years later, in the same area, that "the hole" was bulldozed in and this practice of prisoner punishment ceased.

THE LUCID INTERVAL

The lucid interval happened over forty years ago in the emergency room.

It was a soft, early summer evening and I was the emergency room doctor on-call. It was an evening of trivia—lacerations, fish hooks in legs, earaches. Then the charge nurse asked me to see a frail elderly woman who, in a puff of wind, had been blown off a curb and struck her head on the edge. She was unconscious when medics arrived at the scene of the accident but then she seemed to wake up.

There was a bruise over the brow of her head and an irregular laceration. When I met her she was perfectly rational and signed the emergency form allowing treatment. I noticed she had slight motor weakness and signs of a serious head injury but there were no other injuries. She was mildly hypertensive and told me she took pills for this (she didn't know the name). Then her pulse became slow and one pupil gradually dilated. X-rays of her skull revealed a fracture under the massive swelling. When she was brought back from the x-ray room she lost consciousness again.

I called the neurosurgeon, the operating room and alerted the anaesthetist.

Her phone number, given in the lucid interval, was rung but failed to reach anyone. We had no other contacts to follow up with as her purse was with the police. We typed and cross-matched her for three units of blood.

Within thirty minutes the neurosurgeon had drilled burr holes into her skull, revealing a subdural hematoma. A large bony flap was cut away and there was a lot of bleeding; the brain was pulped. Clot and brain were sucked away. She went into shock from blood loss. I wrote the order to give the blood and it was pumped into her while we controlled her head bleeding. She died weeks later in hospital.

Before she died, during what we had hoped was her recovery phase, I learned that she and her family were devout religious fanatics. Her family and friends accosted me at the hospital and my office to berate me for giving her blood.

A month later I received notice from a large Toronto legal firm that I thought threatening. It stated that this religious group was taking legal action. I notified my malpractice insurance agency.

It was fortuitous that the dying woman had signed, in her lucid interval, the emergency room sheet authorizing treatment.

I continued to work despite the letters and phone calls from this religious cult. My wife and I had four daughters and things were hectic at home and at work. I had trouble sleeping, my dreams violent, my mood a savage melancholy.

Months later the letters from the Toronto lawyers stopped. The malpractice suit was dropped and my malpractice insurance company's lawyers were paid. My lawyers advised me that I should never give a devout individual a blood transfusion that would contravene with their religious beliefs.

For the next few years I received nasty mail at Christmas and on the anniversary of the woman's death. This sectarian group derided me for my decision to give blood and they condemned my soul to eternal damnation.

Finally the correspondence stopped but not before that lucid interval was branded into my brain.

DOUG'S DILEMMA

My friend and colleague Doug had a problem cow on his ranch at Upper Hat Creek in the foothills of the Coast Mountains. The cow was a four-year-old beef cow, a Hereford with a nasty temper. She was so cantankerous that Doug couldn't dehorn her or drive her into a loading shoot to contain her. The local veterinarian refused to do a manual pregnancy test on her each spring because of her behaviour. She'd kick and chase anyone who came into her paddock and hook with her horns and bite anybody who tried to corral her. The kids and ranch hands named her Nasty. But every spring she was pregnant and always dropped a healthy calf. Despite her rotten personality she had the reputation of being a "good breeder."

Doug was a full-time psychiatrist and a part-time rancher. Nasty, with all her shenanigans, was trying to make him into a full-time rancher and a part-time psychiatrist. I was surprised when Doug asked me, a general practitioner, for a consultation with Nasty; he wanted me to help him with his animal problem. I had some expertise with animals as I helped the local veterinarian with his large animal practice and on occasion, gave anaesthetics to bulls and stallions. I didn't know much about the psyche of large cows and their emotional problems but I was willing to learn.

Nasty's abnormal behaviour was making Doug and his family's life miserable. The cow was constantly harassing them and chasing the kids as they walked through the fields on their way to school. Somehow we had to alter her personality and adjust her interpersonal relationships. This was an example of a non-infectious case of mad cow disease. Talking to the animal, even with a few choice phrases, had no effect on her. An electric cattle prod, essentially shock treatment, had no influence on her even after repeated treatment over a period of a month. Counselling accompanied by electrical stimulation was also not the answer to this cow's problem.

At this time, in the 1970s, the drug of choice for the treatment of paranoid, violent behaviour in humans was the antipsychotic drug, chlorpromazine. It was marketed as the injectable solution but also came in pill form. For cows over a thousand pounds the dose was not known. Whether it was safe to use during a cow's pregnancy or if it would be transmitted into the cow's milk and have an effect on the newborn calf was also not known. We had to experiment by trial and error—go by the seat of our jeans, so to speak.

One Saturday afternoon Doug managed to lasso Nasty and get her snubbed down to a snubbing post. After her violent behaviour had ceased and this huge exhausted animal lay down I managed to inject a double dose of drugs into her rump roast. Within an hour Nasty's personality had noticeably changed and the rope snubbing her was slackened. Then to everyone's surprise she ate a bucket of feed laced with my drug samples of antipsychotic drugs. In twenty-four hours Nasty had become a docile cow and every day she took her oats laced with drugs given by Doug's youngest daughter. Nasty soon became the household's pet cow. As a consultant I continued to supply large samples of antipsychotic drugs from the medical clinic's free drug sample collection.

When we ran short of the antipsychotic drug we experimented by substituting Prozac but it didn't seem to work as effectively. Slowly, over a period of many months, we gradually cut back on Nasty's daily dose of drugs but she was never able to be weaned completely. When we noticed any mood swings in her behaviour we would reinstitute her mood-altering drugs.

We all worked as a team. I supplied the free drugs, with the help of the travelling drug salesman. Nasty produced many laconic cows and easygoing bulls with good personalities. Nasty lived out her life in peace and quiet in the shadows of the Canadian Coast Mountains and became a loved and respected member of Doug's Hereford herd. Best of all, it was never necessary to send Nasty to the abattoir in Ashcroft for palliative care.

Mary's Tomatoes

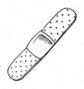

With age, people seem more willing to give out facts about their bodies. When you ask them, "How are you?" you may get more than you bargained for.

Last year in the heat of summer I was walking on Victoria Street, in downtown Kamloops, BC, when a large, grey-haired buxom woman stopped me—she hugged then kissed me on both cheeks. Her husband, a small man, remained ten paces behind her standing in the shade.

"You remember me, Mister Doctor, I'm Mary and that's Joe back there. You delivered all our five kids."

"Oh, yes, now I remember. Just how are you doing, Mary?"

"It's a long story, Mister Doctor. Am I glad to see you, I've really missed you since you retired."

"Thank you, Mary. You haven't been doing well?"

"When I was in hospital with my operations, Mister Doctor, I almost died. See, three scars on my belly."

She lifted her blouse and I could see three new scars, one

paramedian and two vertical on the left side of her abdomen.

"Those are large scars, Mary."

"I really missed you in the hospital. Your friend, the surgeon, I think he was your partner, cut me here, cut me there and after he cut me up and down—three times he cut me."

"I'm so sorry, Mary. What was wrong?"

"Mister Doctor, I almost died. Even the priest thought I was a goner. He gave me my last rites. All the kids was crying in my four-bed hospital ward. It was way past visiting hours too. Even Joe came to see me."

"Sounds bad, Mary."

"I got a tangled bowel, Mister Doctor. It wasn't no cancer neither, 'just a simple bowel obstruction,' the doctor said. Can you believe it?"

"You saw the surgeon?"

"Yes, Doc, your doctor friend cut some bad bowel out of me. Some even had got rotten and I got a bad fever. He hooked my bowel back onto my skin—'a colostomy,' he said. I stayed in the hospital 'til I started passing gas onto my skin. It felt funny, Doc, farting into a big bag. Then your friend he sent me home after he took most of my stitches out."

"He discharged you from hospital?"

"That's right, Mister Doctor. You know Joe, he's got a bad back and he didn't dig my garden and he didn't plant my tomato plants like I told him. When I got home the plants were all wilty-like and Joe was lying and moaning on the couch. I had to do something, Doc."

"What did you do, Mary."

"I done a bad thing, Mister Doctor. I dug the garden with my spade and planted all my tomato plants that evening."

"You did what?"

"I almost finished planting and was pounding my tomato stakes in the ground when everything in my belly came apart. Then I fell down on the plants and lay on the ground. Your friend, the surgeon, got real mad when I came back to the hospital. He said I had 'dehissed.' Would you believe my guts spilled out of me?"

"Did you have to go back for surgery, Mary?"

"Yeah, they washed my belly out good. My belly was full of chicken manure and tomato plants because I fell while hammering my tomato stakes in. Then your friend got real angry when he had to hook me up again. When I woke up about two AM in the recovery room I heard him muttering to himself, 'chicken shit but chicken shit and leaves.' I think he was really mad with me, Mister Doctor."

"I guess you were very sick this time?"

"You said it, Doc. I had two intravenous lines going, one in each arm, and had intensive care for three days and antibiotics by the ton. I almost died. My kids was crying but they never called the priest this time."

"How long did you stay?"

"I was in hospital about two weeks with those big nylon stitches. They held strong—they was thick as my nylon salmon fishing line. Your friend, the surgeon, he left them in for three weeks. When he discharged me the visiting nurses came twice a day, even on Sundays, Mister Doctor. I almost died, those operations were tough."

"What happened then, Mary?"

"About six months later, the surgeon, your friend Doc Gordie, and another nice guy hooked the two ends of my gut together. I've been fine ever since."

"I'm glad you're okay now. Sorry to hear about your problems. I'm meeting your surgeon, Dr. Gordie, right now. We're having lunch together."

"You know, Doc, it's been almost a year. That friend of yours had to cut me three times. But you know, Mister Doctor, he finally got it right."

"It looks like you are doing well now, Mary."

"See you around, Doc, sure do miss you. Tell your surgeon friend I'll bring him some big juicy beefsteak tomatoes next week. They're almost ripe."

Medicine and Mariachi

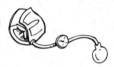

Last September a few members of the Society for Learning in Retirement decided to go to the Mariachi Festival in Guadalajara, Mexico. Twenty of us, including my wife Jesse and my daughter Elizabeth bought our air and theatre tickets for the Degollado Opera House for the Mariachi Festival and decided to fly Horizon Air from Kelowna, BC, to Mexico via Los Angeles. Elizabeth was to act as the Spanish translator for our group of Kelowna-ites while we were in Guadalajara. With three of us in wheelchairs we never thought our group could be mistaken for white-haired terrorists. But in the LA airport our bags were searched, our bodies scanned and our shoes inspected. Then we were searched again, rambo style. US guards herded us along, but the first thing they did was confiscate our water bottles.

The majority of us suffered a little thirst in the California heat but for my friend Constance who has Sjogrens syndrome and is already lacking saliva, sweat and tears, those four hours without water were a serious threat to her general well-being. Medical explanations to the police, attendants and security agents had no effect on the situation—the American regulations said "No Bottles" on planes or in restricted alien passenger holding areas.

In shock and awe we limped and rode our wheelchairs through the many different lines requested by security police. We finally made it to Guadalajara on a short flight and we reached this civil city about three PM. We were loaded with our baggage into three large vans and were taken to the Hotel Frances in downtown Guadalajara, "the city of eternal spring."

I read on the hotel's marquee that it was built in 1610. The foyer was impressive with marble arches and columns and a white and black checkerboard marble floor and magnificent high stained-glass ceilings. The clerks at the desk told us that the hotel had been renovated twenty-nine years before. The ancient elevator worked at times and had been working all day but the night clerk said "it hadn't needed much renovation." Maybe we were in luck as many of the rooms were on the second and third floor. The first to register at the hotel desk were taken up to their rooms in the 1875 vintage cage of the elevator. After the second trip the elevator motor and passenger cage, easily seen in the hobby, started to smoke and smell of burning wire. We didn't need the hotel clerk to warn us of the danger of riding up and down. I wasn't so sure if the Hotel Frances' *el bano* plumbing had been renovated in the twentieth century either. The drains, toilet smells and gurglings could be overwhelming at times.

Unfortunately, one of the women in our group banged her elbow on the stairs while carrying her suitcase up and as a retired MD, known as Doctor X, I was asked for an opinion. I prescribed ice and Advil but two days later large asymptomatic olecranon bursitis appeared. I said, "Give it a bit of tincture of time, won't you please."

The mariachi festival was marvelous. Without realizing it, I had pictured mariachi music as something played only by aging, overweight Mexican trumpeters in tight military tunics and pants tooting away at Mexican dances and political occasions. The thirteenth Encuentro International del Mariachi was a revelation. Part of the performance was with the Guadalajara Philharmonic Orchestra and this was spectacular. The sophisticated orchestras came from countries as diverse as Croatia, Italy and Ireland; even Canada had sent a band. The performance of the Three Mexican Tenors was equal to any production by the Three Tenors or the Three Irish Tenors. After each concert, which was accompanied by dancers, we walked back to the hotel humming the tunes and dancing an abbreviated salsa. Our group was enthralled by the song and dance performed in the restaurants and parks throughout the week.

On the last day of our hotel stay the third medical problem occurred. Verita, a Rubenesque, retired European opera star, had just returned from a shopping spree and joined us for the afternoon happy hour two-for-one margaritas in the hotel's marble foyer. Halfway through my first very strong margarita David, our leader, called me. "Sterling, come quickly. Verita has collapsed on the floor of the bar."

I quickly handed my margarita to David and rushed to Verita's side. She was lying on the cool checkerboard marble floor sweating profusely and clutching her left breast.

"This chest pain is crushing me, Doctor. It goes into my chin and down the inside of my left arm. Do something, my friend."

"How long have you had this pain, Verita? Have you had heart trouble or angina before, do you take nitroglycerine or heart or blood pressure pills?"

"Never, Doctor."

Verita's pulse was rapid but there were no signs of heart failure.

She was hot so I left her lying on the cold marble. I rushed to the desk and asked the clerk to call 911 and an ambulance.

But the clerk replied "Sorry, Doctor, we do not have such a number nor do we have public ambulances in this city. Your friend will have to go in a cab. I'll get a good taxi driver and a new cab. He will be here in a few minutes to take Verita to a very good Mexican cardiac clinic a few kilometres away. Please bring your friend to the entrance and we'll do the rest."

This was the beginning of a wild ride through the crowded streets of Guadalajara during rush hour. My daughter, Elizabeth, went with Verita and her husband, Charles, in the first cab to act as interpreter. My wife and I followed in an older cab. Soon we were following behind a motorcycle cop with his siren blaring and red lights flashing. As we followed the cop down the cleared lane we were joined by curious Mexicans and others who used the car-less traffic lane to get home quickly. The driver of Verita's cab had his head out the window and was screaming in Spanish "esta muriendo, esta muriendo"—she is dying, she is dying. Our beat-up old cab couldn't keep up to the new taxi and the policeman's motorcycle and we fell behind a series of speeding BMWs and Porsches. After about two kilometres we lost sight of the speeding taxi and became hopelessly confused in the city's downtown section. After stopping and asking pedestrians we slowly made our way to the American-style cardiac clinic—we arrived about half an hour later than Verita. Verita had received great service and was being examined by the cardiologist on duty when we arrived. After another three hours, the partly English-speaking emergency room doctor gave us the cardiologist's report.

"Verita is fine and will be able to travel home to Canada tomorrow. Her chest pain has stopped and she is coping well with nitroglycerine."

The complete medical report was given to Verita and with Elizabeth translating I explained the report to Verita and her husband, who had been renamed Chuckito by the Mexicans.

The EKG showed minor T wave changes, nothing definitive. The chest x-ray was negative, the blood count was okay and the cardiac enzymes and electrolytes were normal. The ultrasound of the heart was included in the report and it too was normal. The thallium heart scan was enclosed and regarded as normal. The cardiologist thought Verita had developed a mild angina pectoris attack. His recommendation was to see a cardiologist when she returned to Canada and to continue to use nitroglycerine as necessary. I was impressed with this diagnosis and thought the emergency cardiac clinic was just as good as the emergency cardiac centre at the Kelowna General Hospital, in British Columbia.

The return flight home was uneventful and luckily we didn't have to land in the LA airport. Before we left for home I wrote out an explanation to airport security and airlines personnel that Constance needed to carry water with her at all times because her affliction—Sjogrens disease—demanded it. Constance was allowed to carry a bottle of water through the airports.

Going home we were a little slower as we now had six people riding wheelchairs through the airports but the officials and airport security guards were much more sympathetic on the return journey.

Perhaps, when travelling in the future, I will give up my credentials and responsibilities to emergencies…and no longer will I be known as Doctor X.

You Never Know

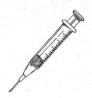

Once I retired from practising medicine, my wife and I started to travel a great deal. Not long ago, in the airport in Raleigh, North Carolina, I struck up a conversation with an older Carolinian contractor. He was going to Creston, British Columbia, to build a straw bale house for his daughter. We were both flying to Toronto before we changed planes, he to Calgary, me to Vancouver. He wanted to build the house soon before he "aged out" or the "hay got too wet and moldy," as he put it.

He asked me, "Is all of Canada a cesspool of disease, or just Toronto?" He had brought paper masks to use in the Toronto airport; they were at the top of his carry-on bag. They were accessible in case of an emergency illness or a new epidemic of SARS or avian flu. "When should I put my mask on," he asked me. "In the plane, deplaning in customs or when I transfer from Toronto to the flight to Calgary?"

I told him, "If you put the mask on in the plane you could be mistaken for a terrorist. This would alert the Air Canada security rent-a-cop. It might be wiser to save your masks for the return flight to Toronto."

"Alright, I'll leave the masks in my case 'til I get to Calgary." Then he said, "Is there mad cow disease in Alberta? The newspapers say 'keep away from hamburger.' And is there monkey pox in Creston or is it confined to the prairie dogs in southern Saskatchewan?"

"There are no threats as far as I know. The case in Canada of monkey pox turned out to be chicken pox," I said.

"What a relief," he said. "I had chicken pox when I was a kid on the plantation. Will this give me immunity now?"

"I'm afraid I can't answer the chicken pox question. I do know there are no prairie dogs in Creston, so you should be safe from this one."

"How about the West Nile virus? My wife packed mosquito netting for the bed and a quart of DEET, to safeguard me. Is it okay to wear shorts in Creston? Heard there are nine different mosquitoes that can transfer this disease from crows to humans. Could be fatal if the infected insects bite your legs at dusk. If there is an outbreak my wife told me 'honey jist ya'all hurry back.'"

"You might want to reconsider and wear shorts while working. Creston can get very hot in summer."

"Yahs sir, I always thought Canadians were a pretty rugged bunch," he said as we parted ways.

"Yes we are hardy; we can survive ice, snow and cold weather. I think the media's hunt for summer diseases is detrimental to our health and to your peace of mind. When hockey starts again in the fall, it'll all be forgotten."

I shook hands with him briskly and wished him a nice day and a safe trip to Creston. As he ascended the airport escalator I noticed him wiping his right hand with his hanky.

ALABAMA

WILLIE'S JOLLIFICATION

In 1980 the US Army and the US Health Development Corporation recruited me to look after the medical needs of the people of Perry County and the cadets of Marion Military Institute. We left BC and moved to Alabama where I practised medicine and my wife, Jessie, ran the clinic.

Sheriff Willie was a criminologist, psychologist, ex-football player and a good friend. He had many layers to his large body. Everyone in the state of Alabama expected Willie to play in the National Football League when he graduated from the University of Alabama. Willie had been a starter, at guard, for coach Bear Bryant and the Crimson Tide football team in Tuscaloosa. When Willie graduated and all the shouting and hoopla was over, he came home to be a cop, to fish and to eat fried chicken and hush puppies—they were his favourites. Catfish was his brain food, turnip greens and fried okra his vitamins. Willie was six foot four, weighed over three hundred pounds and was smart.

Willie was always smiling; his teeth were white except for two gold, false, central upper incisors. His arms were huge, make no mistake. Willie could be formidable when yielding his nightstick but usually he was guileful and spoke with a laugh.

Willie's car was a big 'ole Ford. Everyone knew Willie's car because it had a peculiar sunken look on the driver's side. The shocks on the car were gone on the left and the relaxed springs sat on the front and rear axles.

Willie's peaked cop's cap was always awry and jauntily perched on wooly hair over his right ear. When Willie was driving into the sun the bill of the cap would shade his eyes evenly due to the car's list to the driver's side.

The seats on the left side of the vehicle were torn. Coiled broken springs pushed through the fabric on the back seat. Prisoners complained that the broken springs could "pinch your ass." Willie never did get the seat replaced. A prisoner's sudden cry of pain while sitting in the back seat would evoke a belly laugh from him.

I got to know Willie really well one Friday night at the county hospital emergency room. About eight PM a nineteen-year-old seamstress named Laetitia was brought to the emergency room. She'd been in a knife fight. A big older woman named Mary Ellen brought her to the hospital in her car. The nurse in the ER called Willie then me.

"Doc, we got trouble. A nineteen-year-old, named Laetitia, is here. She's seriously injured with a butcher knife stuck in the right upper quadrant of her belly. There's a crowd of her teenage friends milling around the parking lot looking for trouble. They are holy rollers from the downtown Primitive Evangelical Church. Willie should be here soon. Laetitia's vital signs are good and she's not bleeding much."

"Okay, I'll be right down."

I hurried to the hospital and parked beside Willie's car by the entrance to the ER car park.

"Evening, Doc, we may have a little dust-up with the crowd. They're religious folk but don't expect a heap of trouble," said Willie.

"Hi Willie, hi nurse. Didn't expect to see you here, Mary Ellen," I said.

I'd known Mary Ellen for a few years. She was chief seamstress in the Levy textile plant making tracksuits and jeans. I'd delivered her last three kids. She was a marvel, working full-time and raising six children, mostly by herself. Jethro, her ex, had taken off. She hauled water to her shack, dressed the children, and made sure the kids won academic awards each year. Mary Ellen was robust and very strong.

"What happened?" I asked.

"Well, Doc, this here Laetitia waltzed into my kitchen and said 'no count Jethro' was living with her. She accused me of spreading rumours about town and putting hexes on her and Jethro. I didn't know what she was talking about and told her so. Then she comes at me with a butcher knife. I twisted her arm over and forced the knife into her big belly and then drove her down here. That's it, Doc—she didn't bleed much."

"Mary Ellen, you better stay here in the hospital close to Willie until this rumble is over. I'm going to examine Laetitia on the stretcher, here in the hall."

Laetitia's blood pressure and pulse were okay but I could see the butcher knife sticking out of her belly. As I was checking the knife, I heard a scream and a wail. A huge woman, Laetitia's mother, charged me like an Angus cow. She was shouting, "my baby, my baby." She was running full tilt when she hit me from behind. The nurse had failed to put the brakes on the stretcher and suddenly all three of us were riding down the hall. We hit the distant wall with a crash. I could feel the knife handle under my chest. The mother was on top of me and her huge breast had shoved my head into Laetitia. My sharp elbow scrunched against the mother's nose. I was released as the woman got off me but the knife had been driven deeper into Laetitia and she was screaming.

A chest x-ray revealed a collapsed lung on the right side. IVs were started and I inserted a chest tube in her right chest to release the trapped air. I called the air ambulance in from Tuscaloosa to come and pick up the patient.

While I was phoning I heard hymns and chanting: "God Rest in Jesus," "Follow the Drinking Gourd," "Swing Low Sweet Chariot" and many other old-time slave songs with a syncopated beat. Laetitia's friends had come into the hospital and ER. They lay rolling on the floor and singing in unison much like the "wave" at a football game. The place was bedlam. Willie and the nurses and I tried to reason with these holy rollers. We asked them to leave but to no avail.

Finally, Willie got his nightstick, and laughing and singing with them he grabbed each one by the collar and lifted them off the floor. Then he whacked each one, in turn, on the butt with his club. We all helped propel these religious zealots out the double doors of the hospital emergency room exit.

"Now you folks better git lost," said a laughing Willie, "before I lose my cool and really whup ya'll."

When the helicopter had evacuated Laetitia to Druid City Hospital in Tuscaloosa, Willie, the charge nurse and I went to the hospital cafeteria for coffee. The nurse and I just had coffee but Willie couldn't resist the cook's offer.

"Here, Willie, jist fixed you a big bowl of chicken 'n dumplins, biscuits, fried okra and newly baked apple pie. There's plenty, enough for seconds."

GOUCH!

When practising medicine in Dixieland it helps to have the right words or at least know the meaning in Alabamese, the language of the rural folks. Their speech is colourful and descriptive but their geographical knowledge is poor. When they learned that I was a Canadian doctor from British Columbia some of the locals asked me, "Is that place across the water?" or "Ain't that some place in South America?" The most common question was, "Don't you Colombians grow a lot of pot and coke?"

"Just pot," I said. "It's called BC bud and no coke just coca-cola."

"Oh, you mean coke-colaa, Doc."

At first I used to seek the help of my nurse, Wanda. She was a lively and outspoken African American and got a lot of joy from the crazy questions asked and the colourful expressions used. Sometimes even she was stumped in our medical clinic in Marion, Alabama. On Thursdays from noon to 2:30 PM we used to go to the Venereal Disease Clinic to look after the poor afflicted people. Many of the problems were common but large mommas and a bro or two had a unique way of describing their conditions.

"Hi Doc, shore glad to see you. Ah needs help bad, Doc. My nature done deserted me and that's for sure. Doc, I needs a shot before my new wife takes off."

"What kind of a nature shot is that, Joe?"

"Doc, I just had my seventieth birthday and haven't been able to get it up for two weeks come this Saturday night."

At this time Wanda interjected, "Joe's wife died about a year ago and he's just married a young woman. Doctor, he wants a shot of testosterone for his impotence. He usually gets a prescription and brings it back here and I give him a couple of cc's in his backside. He won't take no for an answer."

Against my better judgement I wrote out the prescription for testosterone and gave it to him.

"Thanks, Doc, and if she done gets pregnant then I'll name the boy after you for sure. Shore do 'preciate it."

The next case was forty-year-old Jean Jones, a diabetic woman who complained "Doc, ah's gotta itchy monkey. This is driving me and Earl crazy; do something, Doc. My new man Earl, he got somethin' too. Ah don't know if I give it to him or he done give it to me. Doc, maybe we's playing catch with it, uh?"

Wanda's definition of a monkey was either the vagina or the labia or both.

"Mrs. Jones, please go into the examining room and we'll take a look with a speculum. There is a sheet in there to cover yourself. If Earl has a penile discharge he better come in to the VD Clinic, too."

"Doc, you ain' goin' to use that cold speclum, are you? Please Doc, warm it up and Earl, he don't like doctors. They's always fixin' to give him a shot of penicillin. He drips a lot from his faucet, leaky-like. And Doc, when you feelin' around for my fire ball, please don't mash my belly too hard."

Wanda informed me that "fire ball" meant fibroids and "to mash" meant to "palpate the abdomen firmly."

"Yes, Mrs. Jones, we'll warm the speculum. I won't mash you hard. Please insist that Earl comes in tomorrow."

After taking a series of slides and wet preps we determined that Mrs. Jones had thrush, chlamydia, and gonorrhea as well as diabetes. After a series of treatments her sexually transmitted diseases had been cured and her diabetes were under control. About three months later Mrs. Jones again appeared with the old refrain, "Say Doc, ah's got an itchy monkey again but Earl's thing's okay for now."

Cawthorn was a great African American always full of fun. He had a wealth of expressions that were very funny. Cawthorn suffered from big toe problems, same as his dad. Early one morning he hobbled into the medical clinic with a swollen, red, painful right big toe.

"Laudy Doc, I never slept a wink last night. Ah's had toe trouble off and on for months. Usually takes a lot of Aspirin but that don't help none last night. Please fix me up, Doc, won't you?"

"Cawthorn, you have arthritis in your big toe. I'll do a blood test and then I'm going to freeze your toe and suck out some fluid from your toe joint; it's probably full of uric acid crystals. I'll give you some new pills that will cure the problem."

"Crystals in my big toe, Doc? They don't shatter none do they? And here ah always figured ah had the gouch."

No interpretation of this disease needed. "Gouch" says it all.

Bubba Biscuit

Bubba was a good 'ole boy from LA—Lower Alabama. He had been raised on a farm near Foley and played football for the Foley Red Devils. After graduation from high school, Bubba won a football scholarship to Auburn University. Bubba was six foot two inches and on his eighteenth birthday weighed three hundred pounds. He was a sweet farm boy through and through. He registered at Auburn U in the department of agriculture and was a proud "Aggie."

His real name was Llewelyn Jones but all his friends called him Bubba. In his final year in high school he was renamed Bubba Biscuit to distinguish him from the other two Bubbas on the team. He got the name Biscuit because he could often be heard to mutter, "well butter my butt and call me biscuit." All his classmates followed his wish.

I got to know Bubba one Saturday in late September. Bubba was a lineman for the Auburn junior varsity football team, the freshmen team. Auburn was playing the cadets at Marion

Military Institute (MMI) in the division two, national college league. I was MMI's regular team doctor but also acted as the Auburn junior varsity team doctor when their Doc didn't show for the game. The football cadets were tougher than pine knots.

The army bands were playing and the cheerleaders chanting and making their moves on the sidelines this bright sunny afternoon. Finally the coin was tossed and play began. Home field was a good one and the stadium was full—about six thousand spectators. The cadets had a good team. Their two stalwarts were Dwight Stone, a running back, and Obadiah Thomas, a defensive end and tight end on the offence. He played both ways and usually played the whole game.

Stone was a big, tough fullback and went on to play in the NFL for the Pittsburgh Steelers. Thomas was six feet eight inches tall and weighed 280 pounds. He went on to play for the University of Alabama under coach Bear Bryant. Both were African Americans and exceptionally fit and strong.

These two men physically manhandled Bubba Biscuit that afternoon. Halfway through the third period Bubba declared, "I'm hotter than a tied-up dawg" as he jogged to the bench. The cadets were well in the lead when Bubba finally returned to his guard position to face Thomas once again.

In the first play of the fourth quarter Thomas drove Bubba back and then pushed him down. There was a cry and Bubba clutched his right shoulder as he lay on the ground. As the team doctor, I rushed onto the field with the medics and the stretcher. When I removed his jersey and his massive shoulder pads I could see Bubba had a dislocated right shoulder. We put him on a stretcher and walked him to the ambulance; with every step Bubba let out a holler and chewed his tobacco more vigorously. By the time we placed him in the ambulance the four stretcher-bearers were groaning, as were the springs on the ambulance.

"Get rid of that chewing tobacco before you drown yourself," I said.

"Okay Doc, but I'll need a couple Styrofoam cups to park it. I got a wad in my cheek that would choke a horse."

Finally we arrived at the small Perry County hospital. The x-rays showed an anterior shoulder dislocation on the right but no fracture. Now the work would begin. I gave him a third of a grain of morphine and injected five milligrams of valium into his vein. I took off my right shoe and put my unshod heel in his axilla in preparation for the reduction. The nurse trickled in a little more morphine and valium into the intravenous tubing as I started to pull on his right arm and push with my right heel, maintaining a steady traction. The sweat poured from me and Bubba's groans became louder and louder. I had used this ancient Hippocratic method of reducing dislocated shoulders many times before but this was the toughest job of relocating a shoulder that I had ever experienced. Bubba's deltoid muscle was the size of a small pony's backside. The muscle spasm in his shoulder was phenomenal. After what seemed like an hour of steady traction there was a satisfying thump, then a "thank Gawd" from Bubba.

"I was kinda worried about you, Doc, and my shoulder too. When that sucker popped in it felt sooo good. Thanks for the Kleenex and the cool wipe to my forehead, nurse. Didn't mean to be a baby. Shore do 'preciate it. Can I get up now, please? I need to pee over a ten-rail fence. I expect I'll be good enough to go home on the team bus?"

"I'll put a collar and cuff-type of sling on you and give you some pain pills. You'll need a great deal of physical therapy before playing again. Be sure to check with the team doctor next week."

About a month later I received a card at my office in Marion from Llewelyn Jones of Opelika, AL. The card read, "Thank ya'll, I'm back at practice today. Been feeling lost as a dog in tall weeds. Now I got my appetite back for fried chicken, grits and biscuits. Getting more strength to do my exercises."

The card was signed "Your friend, Llewelyn Jones (Bubba Biscuit)."

No Coloured Waiting Rooms Here

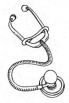

During the time I worked in the deep south of the USA, from 1980–1989, it was common for waiting rooms in clinics outside the larger cities to be segregated. The federal laws of 1964 and 1965 abolished Jim Crow laws of segregation but in rural Alabama these laws were still in effect among the local people. Brown, black and yellow people waited in one waiting room while Caucasian people waited in a different waiting room. The water fountains, toilets and sinks were also colour-coded. In one doctor's office that I visited years ago, the African American people were only allowed to visit the doctor after five PM and their entrance was off the back lane by the "black toilet."

When I went to work for the federally funded Health Development Corporation and the US Army in Marion, Alabama, my wife and I set a precedent in designing our new medical offices. No colour-coded waiting rooms or ice-water fountains or flush toilets and no back lane entrances for African American patients. All people could come and go, at any time, as they wished.

One Monday around noon in September 1982, I received a frantic call from a grade one teacher. This teacher explained that she was supervising the school's cafeteria when she noticed that a six-year-old girl, neatly dressed with her hair in corn rows, eating her lunch, had "an earthworm coming, yes, a worm coming out of her nose."

I explained to the teacher that the worm was not an earthworm but a common intestinal roundworm called *Ascaris*. The woman screamed in reaction to this. I waited until she was silent and then said to her, "Miss, please put on a pair of rubber gloves and clear the mouth of any food, particularly pieces of steak. Then gently pull the worm out from her nose. Some of the rural people using outhouses have basic practices: they think they can lure the worm out of the intestines of their children by having their kids keep a piece of steak in their mouth. They hope the worms will be attracted to the meat and come out their mouth."

After my advice I heard more screaming from the teacher.

"Ma'am, Ma'am, are you okay? Please, just bring the child to the clinic with her mother, now. Do you understand?"

I heard a sob and then, "Yes, Doctor—I'll bring Mary right away, but her mother won't be able to come."

"Okay, I'll tell the nursing staff that Mary is coming."

Every second Monday of each month at one o'clock PM I always saw a wealthy, older white woman, Miss Magdalena, for her monthly appointment. She had a blue rinse to her hair and had a large buffant. Townspeople said, "The higher the hair the closer to God." In this case it was true as she was always quoting from the scriptures and gesturing with her hands. Magdalena had a two-carat diamond on her left ring finger and a one-carat on her right hand. Her rings flashed brightly in my sun-filled waiting room.

That afternoon Mary and Magdalena arrived in the waiting room at the same time. The nurse called me, explaining that there was a problem and to come to the waiting room right away. When I entered the waiting room Magdalena stood up and spoke loudly.

"Doctor, I have a one o'clock appointment the second Monday of each month. Doctor, you do know I have Blue Cross, Blue Shield Alabama insurance, which entitles me to full care. Furthermore, I do not want to wait beside that coloured child with a worm coming out her nose. It is revolting. Yes, disgusting, Doctor. The other, older doctors here have segregated waiting rooms, why can't you?"

"Calm down, Ms. Magdalena. I'll see you in ten minutes but first I will see Mary. Our policy is to have open, non-segregated waiting rooms. We try and deal with everyone fairly. I hope you understand?"

I ushered the little girl and her schoolteacher into my examining room past Miss Magdalena.

"I may have to take my health problems to Selma if this keeps up," muttered Magdalena as I brushed past.

In my examining room I explained to the teacher that the roundworm *Ascaris lumbricoides* was a common parasite amongst anyone who used privies. I quickly put on a pair of rubber gloves and slowly pulled a twelve-inch roundworm from Mary's nostril. My nurse smoothly put it in a jar to be pickled in formalin and sent to the pathologist in Selma.

I looked over to the teacher's pale face and quickly found a chair for her to sit down on before she fainted. I explained that, "The treatment is a single oral dose of medicine called piperazine and it is safe for children. The problem is that all the children in the family must be treated in order for this to be effective—

please tell the mother to contact me for follow-up. I will phone a prescription into College City Drugs. If the parents can't pay, the cost will be charged to the clinic."

"Yes, doctor."

"You and Mary can go back to school after picking up the prescription at the drug store. Remember, if you come across kids chewing on cuds of steak please realize that the parents are trying to entice the worms out of the intestine. Just have the kids spit out the pieces of steak but keep your eyes peeled for roundworms."

Miss Magdalena did come back to our clinic but always arrived at 12:45 PM to insure that she would be the first patient seen in the clinic after lunch. I did not mention the problems of *Ascaridae* in the schools to Miss Magdalena—I didn't want to open up "a bag of worms," so to speak.

I'm glad to say that slowly, after a few years, these racial problems in my office were overcome. The ice-water fountains and flush toilets of our clinic in the small city of Marion, Alabama, were never colour-coded. They were free to all regardless of skin colour.

Jake the Lineman

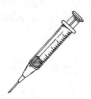

In the summer of 1989 the insects were buzzing. The crape myrtle and rhododendrons were blooming in the sultry heat of a burnt August. The bushes were droning with hornets, wasps and bees. Jake, a lineman for Alabama Power, in Perry County, arrived at a downed, hot power line beside the giant magnolia tree on the edge of town.

Jake had been allergic to wasp stings since he was in high school. On this Monday morning Jake had taken over a new Ford Alabama Power truck but he had forgotten to transfer his Epi-Pen emergency kit to the new vehicle's glove compartment. He was working without injectable adrenaline close at hand. When Jake realized he was without his EpiPen he felt anxious but the high tension wire on the side of the road was hot and posed an immediate threat to passersby. After parking his vehicle he placed red stanchions around the dangerous wire.

Then he rolled up the sleeves of his flannel shirt and strapped on his climbing boot spurs. Jake managed to get to the top of the power pole and had just clipped the dangerous piece of copper close to the insulator when a cloud of wasps attacked. Quickly he climbed down the pole. Slapping at these insects he fled to the safety of his truck cab but not before he had received multiple stings to his neck and arms. Jake started to wheeze and knew he had to get medical help fast. He roared down the road to the clinic, a mile away. His breath became more laboured by the second.

He pulled up at the front door of the Perry Clinic, left the motor running and stumbled to the entrance, collapsing against the glass door. Geraldine, the office manager, spotted him and rushed to his aid, followed by Wanda, my nurse, with the stretcher; I was right behind them. Jake was lying on the white sidewalk cyanotic. His nose, lips and nail beds were a deep blue. As they say in Alabama he was covered with "whelps" from the stings.

Jake was a chunky guy, well over two hundred pounds. While Wanda held his head I grabbed him by his belt and lifted him onto the stretcher. Immediately I felt pain and something rip in my right groin and I heard a gurgle. There was no time to lose if I wanted to save Jake. While wheeling the patient into our treatment room Wanda noticed Jake's medical alert bracelet. It said "I am allergic to wasp and bee stings."

Wanda started the flow of oxygen by mask. I gave 0.5 cc of 1:1000 adrenaline in his arm, subcutaneously. I inserted an intracatheter into a large vein in his massive forearm and started an IV with one litre of normal saline; hydrocortisone and benadryl were given immediately by a "push" into the IV tubing. There was little improvement over the next few minutes so then I gave him 0.25 cc of adrenaline directly into his vein. The results were amazing: his colour returned to normal and his wheeze and air hunger stopped but he was still covered in sweat.

Wanda, our colourful African American nurse, broke the

tension with one of her Alabama expressions.

"Jake looks like he been rode hard and put away wet."

"I'll go park his truck out front and phone his wife now that he looks better," said Geraldine. "She'll want to come down here, I'm sure."

"Good," said Wanda. "Boy, but he was sure 'jammed up and jelly tight' when we first got to him. I'll get a towel now and wipe him off. Look here at all the wasps Jake killed—they're hidden in the folds of his shirt. I'll put some in a test tube for identification and label them."

"Thanks everyone. Good thinking, Wanda. This was a team effort," I said smilingly. "You feeling better now, Jake?"

"Yes sir, Doc. But shore needs to take a leak 'bout now."

"Sure, Jake, but take the IV bag of fluid with you when you go. Please don't disrupt the intravenous line. The toilet is just around the corner but I could bring you a urine bottle if you want."

"Thanks, Doc, but no pee bottles for me."

Just before we closed the office I checked Jake over again and he said he was "feeling great."

After the emergency was over, I had time to notice the discomfort and fullness in my groin, which continued to increase throughout the day. I had a large, complete inguinal hernia on the right side. The next day, Dr. Sam, my surgeon in Selma, showed me a large, fine-mesh plastic cloth that he would use in my hernia repair.

"Doc, I'm going to sew this mesh into your rupture repair. Your groin will be so tight not even a boll weevil can get through. I'm really going to 'mesh' you up," said Dr. Sam with a belly laugh.

Before Jake returned to work I referred him to a specialist at the University of Alabama. Jake took the insect samples of the wasps that stung him to the professor. Then the immunologist at the university in Birmingham made special shots for him. The venom of these wasps was diluted and he was given increasing doses of his special, specific vaccine as allergy shots. Every week Jake came to Perry Clinic and we gave him these specially made injections. I always had a syringe full of adrenaline close at hand.

After this incident, Jake always carried a small EpiPen kit with him in his hip pocket, just in case. In the other hip pocket he carried a round plug of chewing tobacco for real emergencies.

Blue Jeebies

A short while ago my wife was going through old office files from my Alabama medical clinic and came upon a letter from the local garbage collector. His name, appropriately, was Taker. Taker was a tall, angular man, part African American and part Cherokee. He was born on Buckaloo Mountain in eastern Alabama in a home close to the house where Joe Louis, the former heavyweight boxing champion of the world, was born and raised.

My wife gave me the letter and said, "Isn't this a gem?"

The letter touched me. It was the answer to a medical bill I had sent to Taker. The letter was printed on unlined, poor quality paper dated August 16, 1982. Attached was a cheque for the full amount. Here is the printed letter in part—the letter's contents were obviously written by the town letter writer.

Dr Haynes:

Dear Sir,

It was so nice to hear from you...

I liked you as a man immensely and your services were most satisfactory. Please accept the check—your fees were very modest and it could have been the other way around.

Have it as a token of my appreciation for the help you gave me in my time of *great need*.

May God bless you with all the better things of life is my solemn wish always.

Very respectfully,

(signed) Taker

Taker was an honest, God-fearing Baptist, who had a dark drinking habit. The booze was purchased from the bootlegger in the alley just behind the Piggly Wiggly Groceteria.

He would start drinking moonshine after work on Friday and would continue imbibing until the stroke of midnight Saturday. Taker would sober up on Sunday. Sometimes, he'd miss the morning service at Ezekiel Primitive Baptist Church but he'd never miss the evening worship. He'd be prepared for the heat, flies, smell and heavy lifting that would begin seven AM Monday morning when he started working for the county.

Taker was a redeemer and always prayed in church. Early one Sunday morning in August, Taker came to the county hospital smelling of booze. I was called to see him because he had shot off his big toe with a colt .38 revolver...aptly nicknamed a Saturday night special.

"Ya see, Doc, ah'd been drinkin' since Friday after supper. Ah picked up a gallon of hooch from a Buckaloo Mountain liquor still and the bootlegger said this batch was plenty strong."

"How much did you drink?"

"Me and my buddies drank the whole shebang."

"What happened then?" I asked.

"Must of passed out, my friends took me home. My wife cleaned me up and put me to bed in the spare room."

"What woke you up, Taker?"

"Sometimes I get the blue jeebies. Them voices and visions woke me up. Other times ah get moonshine heebie hexes."

"You mean the DTs."

"Yahs sir, ah gets nervous, Doc. Ah see's things like snakes and hands comin' at me, comin' for to punish me for my evil drinkin' ways. Last night, in the moonlight, I woke up and seen this big black hand and monster thumb coming at me to gouge my eyes out."

"What did you do?"

"Ah found mah pistol, a .38, on the bed table. Ah sat up in bed and that big black right thumb came at me to blind me."

"And then..."

"Ah pushed the safety off, Doc, and I shot that big black thumb right through that long dirty nail."

"You mean you shot your big toe off?"

"You got it right, Doc, you figures real well."

"Taker, I'll have to partially amputate the toe. I'll freeze it first, shouldn't feel a thing. You'll end up with a smaller toe without a toenail."

"Praise to you, in my time of great need. Don't 'spect I'll make that Sunday morning sermon at church. Will I, Doc?"

"If you hurry, Taker, you can make it. Be sure to keep your foot elevated on the pew in church and during the week at home. Please check with me if you have any trouble. The nurse will give you some pain pills. Drop in to see me next Friday and I'll change the dressing. Please keep away from the moonshine until your toe is healed, okay?"

"Okay, and thanks, Doc. Ah's certainly going to pray for ya'll."

Obadiah and Bernice

It was a sad day for me when I read in the Toronto *Globe and Mail* of the death of Coretta Scott King. As a doctor I treated her aging parents for ten years and had come to know her as well.

Obadiah and Bernice King, from Heiberger, Alabama—a hamlet close to Marion—were two patients in my new clinic in Perry County. They were well spoken and as leaders of the black community they endorsed me as their doctor and spread the word that I was an "okay Doc." Their daughter, Coretta Scott King, had been educated at a private missionary school and graduated first in her class at the Lincoln School in downtown Marion. They gave me Coretta's phone number in Atlanta and instructed me to call Mrs. King if either of them developed major health problems. As Obie and Bernice were both in their eighties I phoned Atlanta quite regularly. Mrs. Coretta Scott King always had time to talk to me about her folks and life in Marion even though I knew she was busy lobbying in Washington to have the third Monday of every January set aside as a national holiday, "Martin Luther King Day."

Coretta Scott King was labelled by the press as cold and at times calculating but I never found that to be true. Whenever I phoned Atlanta her voice was soft and slow. She was always focussed and concerned. When her mother, Bernice, developed a malignancy, Mrs. Scott was moved. The next day she arranged for her mother to be transported to Emory's University Hospital in Atlanta for treatment.

Although Obie and Bernice were my regulars they only came when they had a serious medical problem. They were a special pair. Obie was a small, sinewy, tough old man who still ran a small "Gro" in Heiberger. He was honest and wouldn't put up with any nonsense. He stored a .44 revolver under the counter of his grocery store, so he said, and practised shooting targets with the gun every day at dawn. Nobody messed with Obie. He always asked for an appointment for nine o'clock in the morning and was always with Bernice. He would get very impatient if he wasn't seen immediately and sometimes would "pitch-a-fit" if there was a delay. He demanded to be seen first until one day in my office Bernice hit Obie with her purse and demanded that she be seen first.

"Obie, you're always barging in ahead of me and speaking for me. I can speak for myself. You get out of here until I've talked to the doctor." After this episode Bernice seemed to be in charge and I always saw her first despite Obie's scowls.

Bernice, at eighty-five years, was still a tall, beautiful woman, eloquent in her speech but just as feisty as Obie. We became good friends.

The Scotts always applauded me for having the first non-segregated medical clinic in Marion. Everyone, black and white, was free to use our flush toilets and to drink ice water from our water fountains. During the summer heat all fifty waiting room chairs were in use—everyone enjoyed the air-conditioned waiting room and the daily gossip. As a local African American leader, Obie always knew when I'd made house calls in the black section of Marion.

Obie and Bernice were very proud of their middle daughter Coretta, and Martin, their son-in-law. When I think of the Scotts, I often think of Martin Luther King's speech, "I Have a Dream," which he gave to over two hundred thousand people at the Lincoln Memorial Center in Washington in 1963. His speech exemplified the philosophy of all the Scotts: "I have a dream that one day this nation will rise up and live out the true meaning of its creed. We hold these truths to be self evident, that all men are created equal..."

When I decided to retire from medicine and return to British Columbia, Obie brought my wife and me watermelons galore and Bernice baked us a pound cake. Bernice "hugged my neck" and Obie, aged ninety-two, shook my hand and told me that I was one of the first "whiteys" that he had ever trusted.

Acknowledgements

I would like to thank my family and the women in my life who helped with this collection of stories. Dona Sturmanis, teacher, editor and writer was instrumental in getting me started writing. Later, my daughters Elizabeth and Leslie Haynes helped me to be concise and exact in my writing. Elizabeth was patient with me and did the bulk of the editing of this book. My sweet wife, Jessie, did all a wife could do to help with ideas, transition, context and punctuation of my collection. Vici Johnstone, the publisher of Caitlin Press, made timely suggestions and positive decisions that helped make my book marketable. I am indebted to Erin Schopfer who made constructive suggestions and did the final editing.

Joe McAlister, features editor for Roger Publishing, published the majority of these stories in *The Medical Post*. Joe liked, edited and promoted my work. Naji Naaman, Parisian French publisher, awarded my story, *Divinity*, a "literary honour prize" in a 2008 anthology of prose in French, English and Arabic. For my yarn, "*Doc, We Got a Problem*," the Shuswap Writer's Festival awarded me the Joyce Dunn prize for creative non-fiction. All these people believed in my work and encouraged me. I am indebted to them.

I'm indebted to Dr. John Roberts, archivist, and the staff at the Williams Lake Library who helped me select pertinent archives.

I wish to acknowledge the help and support of the city of Edmonton archivists and Debbie Shoctor, archivist for the Jewish Archives and Historical Society of Edmonton and Northern Alberta. Mrs. Florence Weinlos Soifer, Dr. Harry's niece, was full of facts and stories about the life of her Uncle Harry. Her help and encouragement were exceptional.